**Felix Rietmann**

**ClC-channels and etoposide resistance**

AF061451

Felix Rietmann

# ClC-channels and etoposide resistance

## An experimental study of the neuroendocrine tumour cell line LCC-18

Südwestdeutscher Verlag für Hochschulschriften

**Imprint**

Any brand names and product names mentioned in this book are subject to trademark, brand or patent protection and are trademarks or registered trademarks of their respective holders. The use of brand names, product names, common names, trade names, product descriptions etc. even without a particular marking in this work is in no way to be construed to mean that such names may be regarded as unrestricted in respect of trademark and brand protection legislation and could thus be used by anyone.

Publisher:
Südwestdeutscher Verlag für Hochschulschriften
is a trademark of
Dodo Books Indian Ocean Ltd., member of the OmniScriptum S.R.L Publishing group
str. A.Russo 15, of. 61, Chisinau-2068, Republic of Moldova Europe
Printed at: see last page
**ISBN: 978-3-8381-2530-5**

Zugl. / Approved by: Berlin, Charité, Diss., 2010

Copyright © Felix Rietmann
Copyright © 2011 Dodo Books Indian Ocean Ltd., member of the OmniScriptum S.R.L Publishing group

# Contents

**1 Introduction** — 1
  **1.1 Neuroendocrine tumours** — 1
    1.1.1 Definition and history of the diffuse neuroendocrine system — 1
    1.1.2 Short history of neuroendocrine tumours — 2
    1.1.3 Features of the diffuse neuroendocrine system — 3
    1.1.4 Epidemiology of neuroendocrine tumours — 3
    1.1.5 Classification of gastroenteropancreatic neuroendocrine tumours (GEP-NETs) — 4
    1.1.6 Clinical presentation — 5
    1.1.7 Treatment — 5
  **1.2 Drug resistance** — 6
    1.2.1 ATP-binding cassette transporters — 7
    1.2.2 pH and drug resistance — 7
    1.2.3 pH regulation of intracellular compartments — 8
    1.2.4 V-ATPase and ClC-channels in cancer and drug resistance — 12
  **1.3 Etoposide** — 13
  **1.4 Aim of this study** — 13

**2 Materials and methods** — 15
  **2.1 Materials** — 15
  **2.2 Methods** — 15
    2.2.1 Cell culture and generation of resistant cell lines — 15
    2.2.2 Quantification of acridine orange fluorescence from acidic compartments — 16
    2.2.3 Cell proliferation assay — 17
    2.2.4 Quantitative real time polymerase chain reaction (qPCR) — 18

**3 Results** — 24
  **3.1 LCC-18 Resistant to 1nM concanamycin A** — 24
    3.1.1 Generation and vesicular acidity of LCC-18 resistant to 1nM concanamycin A — 24
    3.1.2 Etoposide sensitivity of LCC-18 resistant to 1nM concanamycin A — 26
    3.1.3 Genetic expression of LCC-18 resistant to 1nM concanamycin A — 27
  **3.2 LCC-18 resistant to 1µM etoposide** — 31
    3.2.1 Generation of LCC-18 resistant to 1µM etoposide — 31
    3.2.2 Vesicular acidity of LCC-18 resistant to 1µM etoposide — 32
    3.2.3 mRNA expression in LCC-18 resistant to 1µM etoposide — 33

**4 Discussion** — 35
  **4.1 LCC-18 resistant to 1nM concanamycin A** — 35
    4.1.1 Vesicular acidity and etoposide resistance — 35
    4.1.2 Gene expression, vesicular acidity and etoposide resistance — 35
  **4.2 LCC-18 resistant to 1µM etoposide** — 37
    4.2.1 Vesicular acidity and etoposide resistance — 37
    4.2.2 Gene expression — 37
  **4.3 Conclusion** — 40

**5 Abstract** — 41

**6 References** — 43

**Appendix** — 47
  List of Abbreviations — 47
  List of Tables and Figures — 48
  Zusammenfassung — 49
  Acknowledgments — 51

# 1 Introduction

## 1.1 Neuroendocrine tumours

### 1.1.1 Definition and history of the diffuse neuroendocrine system

The diffuse neuroendocrine system includes various cell types which share phenotypic properties, but not necessarily an embryological origin. They can be found at different locations in the whole human organism, exhibit endocrine as well as neuronal characteristics and play an important role in the hormonal regulation of organs and the body. They populate the skin, thyroid, lung, thymus, pancreas and gastrointestinal, biliary and urogenital tract, and other locations as well [Klöppel, 2007].

The current notion of the diffuse neuroendocrine system is the result of a complex research history, which dates back to the beginnings of histo-pathological studies in the 19th century. In 1938 the Austrian pathologist Friedrich Freyter (1895-1973) established the first comprehensive concept of the neuroendocrine system. By unifying previous pathological discoveries with his own histological studies of the pancreas and the gastrointestinal tract, he suggested that endocrine cells were scattered individually and in groups throughout the epithelium of human organs and were part of the endocrine system. His hypothesis marked a break with the hitherto accepted theory that organs constituted "compact epithelial bodies" with individual and unique functions and properties. Moreover, he linked the diffuse endocrine system to nervous tissue and thus founded the concept of the diffuse neuroendocrine system as an interface of humoral and nerval regulation of organ functions, notably in the gastrointestinal tract [Champaneria, 2006; Modlin, 2006; Pearse, 1977]. Although Freyter's work constituted a milestone in the understanding of human physiology, it was little recognized in his time and it was only in the 1960s that new efforts were undertaken to establish a comprehensive view of the neuroendocrine system. Based on Freyter's work, the British histochemist A.G.E. Pearse (1916-2003) developed the so-called "APUD" (amine precursor uptake and decarboxylation) system. This acronym was derived from the common biochemical ability of neuroendocrine cells to produce, store and secrete low-weight polypeptide hormones. This functional pattern was mirrored in ultra structural characteristics (see below). Pearse integrated not only

Freyter's diffuse neuroendocrine system into his classification, but also cells of several endocrine organs, including the thyroid and pituitary gland as well as the pancreas, and suggested that all originated embryologically from the neuronal crest [Pearse, 1969].

The enormous progress of research at the end of the 20$^{th}$ century and in the beginning of the 21$^{st}$ century led to an expansion and revision of Pearse's concept. It could be shown that different embryological origins could lead to a neuroendocrine phenotype and, most recently, that inflammation could cause cells to acquire neuroendocrine characteristics, thus linking the immune to the neuroendocrine system. However, there remain many open questions concerning this important regulatory system [Modlin, 2006].

**1.1.2 Short history of neuroendocrine tumours**

In 1907, the German physician Siegfried Oberndorfer (1876-1944) introduced the term carcinoid in order to distinguish a morphologically distinct class of tumours of the small intestine from the more aggressive and more common intestinal adenocarcinomas. Gosset and Masson demonstrated in 1914 that the cells of this tumour contained silver salt reducing (argentaffin) granules and therefore suggested their endocrine origin. This led to the concept of the carcinoid tumour as a neoplasm that contained argentaffin cells and derived from a special cell type in the small intestine, known as Kultchitsky cells. In subsequent years, a characteristic clinical syndrome, including flush, diarrhoea and intermittent bronchoconstriction, could be linked to the carcinoid group of tumours. Furthermore, an association of the symptoms with overproduction of 5-hydroxytryptamine (serotonin) was shown. Tumours with similar clinical and biochemical findings from locations other than the small intestine were discovered and led to a broader definition of carcinoid tumours. A first classification system of carcinoid tumours was introduced by Williams and Sandler in 1963, just as Pearse systematised the neuroendocrine system as the APUD system. However, the term neuroendocrine tumour was not introduced systematically before 1994. It now serves to designate the totality of neoplasm with neuroendocrine features, formerly described in an arbitrary fashion as carcinoid tumours [Williams, 1961; Creutzfeldt, 1996].

## 1.1.3 Features of the diffuse neuroendocrine system

Today, the identification of a neuroendocrine cell relies on morphological, histological and antigenic properties. Neuroendocrine cells are either organised in trabecular clusters or dispersed among other cells. In histological sections, they have uniform nuclei and abundant granular or clear cytoplasm. They may exhibit an affinity to chromium salt and may be able to take up and decarboxylate amine precursors. At an ultra-structural level, they contain cytoplasmic membrane-bound dense-core secretory granules (diameter > 80nm) as well as small clear vesicles (diameter 40–80 nm) that correspond to the synaptic vesicles of neurons. Immunostaining makes their exact identification possible. Their assessment comprises characteristic antigens, which include molecules of the cytosol as well as antigens of secretory vesicles. Among the former group are the neuron-specific enolase and protein gene product 9.5, the latter group notably includes the chromogranines (A, B and C) and synaptophysin. The hormonal content of the secretory granules determines the specific cell type. In the gastrointestinal tract and the pancreas, 15 cell types that produce different hormones can be distinguished [Klöppel, 2007; Rindi, 2004; Plöckinger, 2004; Modlin, 2006].

## 1.1.4 Epidemiology of neuroendocrine tumours

Neuroendocrine tumours are a rare, mostly sporadic disease representing only 0.5% of all malignancies. The incidence accounts for approximately 2/100,000 and has been rising for the last decades, which might mainly be due to improved diagnosis. Neuroendocrine tumours localise preferentially in the gastrointestinal tract (62%) followed by the lung (23%). The peak incidence occurs at the age of 65, with the exception of tumours of the appendix, which occur more commonly under the age of 50. Although they are sporadic in most patients, they can be part of the multiple endocrine neoplasia type 1 syndrome or develop secondary to chronic atrophic gastritis, and a familial risk has been described for several subtypes [Klöppel, 2005]. Generally, the 5-year survival of patients has significantly increased in recent years, though it depends mainly on the stage of the disease at diagnosis. While 93% of patients diagnosed in the local disease stage sur-vive 5 years, the survival decreases to 74% in regional and 19% in metastatic cases [Taal, 2004].

## 1.1.5 Classification of gastroenteropancreatic neuroendocrine tumours (GEP-NETs)

Because of their rarity, until now no structured practice for diagnosis and therapy of GEP-NETs has been developed. However, the World Health Organisation (WHO) recently introduced a revised classification of tumours of the diffuse endocrine system, which was the basis for the development of common diagnostic and treatment guidelines by the European Neuroendocrine Tumour Society (ENETS).

As outlined above, Williams and Sandler developed a first classification of GEP-NETs in 1961. They categorised these tumours by their origin into foregut (stomach, pancreas, duodenum and upper jejunum), midgut (lower jejunum, ileum, appendix, caecum) and hindgut (colon, rectum) tumours with important clinical differences between the three groups. Although this classification has limitations for the current clinical practise, especially concerning the very broad and heterogeneous group of foregut NETs, it is still used for rough characterisation.

The current WHO classification divides endocrine tumours of the diffuse gastroenteropancreatic neuroendocrine system into three categories according to their pathological differentiation:

1. Well-differentiated endocrine tumours with:
    1.1. Benign or
    1.2. Uncertain behaviour at the time of diagnosis;
2. Well-differentiated endocrine carcinomas with low-grade malignant be behaviour;
3. Poorly- differentiated endocrine carcinomas, with high-grade malignant behaviour.

Because of their highly aggressive behaviour, the neoplasms of the third category differ profoundly from those of category 1 and 2 and require a special therapeutic approach [Klöppel, 2007; Plöckinger, 2004].

The European Neuroendocrine Tumour Society proposed in their guidelines a tumour/nodes/metastases (TNM) classification of foregut GEP-NETs and a grading system of digestive NETs based on mitotic counts and the Ki-67 index [Rindi, 2006]. For clinical practise the following table was suggested:

## Criteria for assessing the prognosis of neuroendocrine tumours of the gastrointestinal tract

| Biological behaviour | Metastases | Invasion of muscularis propria[a] | Histological differentiation | Tumour size | Angio-invasion | Ki-67 Index | Hormonal syndrome |
|---|---|---|---|---|---|---|---|
| Benign | - | - | Well differentiated | ≤ 1cm[a] | - | < 2 % | -[a] |
| Benign or low grade malignant | - | - | Well differentiated | ≤ 2cm | -/+ | < 2 % | - |
| Low grade malignant | + | +[b] | Well differentiated | > 2cm | + | > 2 % | + |
| High grade malignant | + | + | Poorly differentiated | Any | + | >30% | - |

[a] Exception: malignant duodenal gastrinomas are usually smaller than 1cm and confined to submucosa
[b] Exception: Benign NETs of the appendix usually invade the muscularis propria

**Table 1:** Criteria for assessing the prognosis of neuroendocrine tumours of the gastrointestinal tract [modified from Klöppel, 2005]

### 1.1.6 Clinical presentation

Depending on their ability to cause a hormone hypersecretion syndrome, neuroendocrine tumours can be divided into non-functioning and functioning tumours. Mainly, two properties determine whether a hormone-related syndrome occurs: the first relates to the tumour's ability to produce biogenic amines; the second addresses the localisation of the tumour, i.e. its ability to secrete a sufficient amount of biogenic amines into the posthepatic circulation. A hormonal hypersecretion syndrome is thus frequently observed in metastatic disease. While poorly differentiated neuroendocrine tumours usually lack hormone activity, various clinical presentations are found in more differentiated neoplasms. Especially foregut neuroendocrine tumours can produce a variety of different hormones, which can cause diverse clinical presentations. Characteristic for serotonin-producing NETs is the so-called carcinoid syndrome characterised by flush, diarrhoea and intermittent bronchoconstriction. Carcinoid heart disease might be associated with this presentation, and, if untreated, heart failure rather than metastatic disease may limit survival [Plöckinger, 2004; Plöckinger, 2005].

### 1.1.7 Treatment

While treatment of GEP-NETs with curative intention relies upon surgical therapy, for patients with metastatic disease several treatment options exist that aim at reduction of symptoms and improvement of response to systemic chemotherapy. These include cytoreductive therapy other than surgery, e.g.

chemoembolisation and local ablative therapy, and biotherapy, which uses derivatives of naturally occurring substances of the body. Generally, neuroendocrine malignancies are less sensitive to chemotherapy than other epithelial tumours; especially well-differentiated GEP-NETs show a very low response to chemotherapeutic drugs due to their low growth rate.

Poorly differentiated GEP-NETs are aggressive tumours that usually present with metastases at time of diagnosis and tend to progress rapidly. Surgery is rarely possible and ineffective even in locally advanced disease due to a high risk of recurrence. Thus, chemotherapy with cisplatin and etoposide constitutes the reference treatment and frequently yields response rates greater than 50%. However, disease control is limited to 8-10 months and median survival amounts to approximately 15 months [O'Toole, 2004; Arnold, 2005; Moertel, 1991]. Especially in these patients, drug resistance constitutes a major problem and it is thus of high interest to develop additional therapeutic strategies.

## 1.2 Drug resistance

Chemotherapeutic treatment of cancer takes advantage of the phenomenon that tumour cells are more sensitive to anticancer drugs than normal cells. This hypersensitivity is presumably due to an enhanced replication rate and increased metabolism. However, a major impediment of anticancer therapy lies in the evolution of drug resistance during treatment. Furthermore, diminished sensiti-vity to the original drug may also extend to a broad class of other drugs, diverse in their structure and target. This acquired multidrug resistance (MDR) constitutes a major challenge to successful chemotherapy of malignant tumours [Simon, Roy, and Schindler, 1994; Simon, and Schindler, 1994].

For the last 35 years, clinical scientists have focused on the assessment of cellular mechanisms that confer drug resistant phenotypes and have revealed an extraordinary diversity of genetic and biologic changes in cancer cells. Studies have investigated either the specific nature and genetic background of the cancer cell itself or the genetic changes that follow toxic chemotherapy. The latter studies are mainly based on the selection of surviving cancer cells in the presence of cytotoxic agents and subsequent analysis of genetic and biological changes in these cells. Generally, drug resistant cells are thought to have one or both of the following features:

An altered susceptibility to the drug, which might be due to alterations in cell cycle, alterations of the drug target, increased repair of DNA damage, reduced apoptosis or altered metabolism of drugs.

Lower intracellular drug concentrations. This might be achieved by decreased uptake of water-soluble drugs, energy-dependent efflux of hydrophobic drugs or sequestration of the drug in intracellular vesicles [Szakács, 2006; Raghunand, 1999; Stavrovskaya, 2000; Simon, Roy, and Schindler, 1994; Simon, and Schindler 1994].

### 1.2.1 ATP-binding cassette transporters

The most commonly encountered mechanism of drug resistance is the increased energy-dependent efflux of hydrophobic drugs mediated by adenosine triphosphate (ATP) binding cassette transporters. The latter constitute a large group of conserved proteins, which are named after their distinctive ATP-binding cassette domain. Generally, they translocate solutes across cellular membranes. The human genome contains 48 genes encoding the ABC transporters, which have been divided into 7 subfamilies labelled A-G. Their substrates range from naturally occurring biological compounds to chemotherapeutic drugs, and it has become increasingly evident that they play a pivotal role in host detoxification and protection of the body against xenobiotics. At least 12 members of the large family of ABC transporters are known to be involved in multidrug resistance of cells maintained in tissue culture. Most abundantly expressed in drug resistant cells are ABCB1, ABCC1 and ABCG2, also named P-glycoprotein (Pgp), multidrug resistance associated protein 1 (MRP1), and breast cancer resistance protein 1 (BCRP1), respectively [Szakács, 2006]. Although these drug efflux pumps are generally considered to be cell surface localized, recent studies found evidence that sub-cellular localization might also play a role in drug resistance. Residing in intracellular compartments, these proteins may sequester drugs actively away from their cellular targets [Rajagopal, 2003].

### 1.2.2 pH and drug resistance

Particular pH properties of cancer tissue as well as chemical properties of anticancer drugs gave rise to another hypothesis of acquired multidrug resistance, called the "ion trapping hypothesis" or "protonation, sequestration and secretion model", which is based on the following principle [Atlan, 1998; Raghunand, 2000]:

Chemotherapeutic regimes employ a huge variety of agents, which can be divided by their chemical properties under physiological conditions into weak-acid, neutral and weak-basic drugs. Weak-base drugs ionize in solution into positively charged, protonated molecules and uncharged, unprotonated forms. While physiological membranes of cells are fairly permeable for the uncharged forms, the charged molecules cannot cross the lipid layer. The relatively high permeability of the plasma membrane to uncharged drugs leads to equilibration of unprotonated molecules on both sides of the membrane, while charged drugs are supposed to concentrate on the more acid side of the membrane, which leads to greater total drug concentration in acidic compartments [Atlan, 1998; Raghunand, 1999; Raghunand, 2000]. Acidified organelles may, thus, protonate chemotherapeutic drugs and sequester them away from the nucleoplasm and cytosol. Subsequently, the drugs may be secreted from the cell through the normal pathways of vesicular traffic and secretion. Since the extent of partitioning of weak-base drug molecules across the plasma membrane of a tumour cell depends on the pKa of the drug and the pH gradient across the cellular membranes, an alkaline-inside pH gradient across the plasma membrane in combination with an enhanced acidification of intracellular vesicles in tumour cells would exert a protective effect upon the cells from weak-base drugs [Atlan, 1998; Raghunand, 1999; Raghunand, 2000; Schindler, 1996; Roos, 1978; Simon, Roy, and Schindler, 1994].

The emergence of the ion-trapping hypothesis therefore underlines the importance of understanding the pH regulation of intracellular vesicles in tumour cells, as these compartments might be able to contribute to resistance to chemotherapy.

### 1.2.3 pH regulation of intracellular compartments

*1.2.3.1 Vacuolar adenosine triphosphatase (v-ATPase)*

Acidification of intracellular vesicles is driven by a family of ATP-dependent proton pumps known as vacuolar ($H^+$)-ATPases. They reside within the lipid bilayer of organelles and acidify the lumen by active transport of protons [Nishi, 2002; Sun-Wada, 2004]. Acidification of intracellular compartments plays an important role in a large number of cellular processes, which include among others the regulation of endo- and exocytic pathways and recycling, sorting and distribution of cellular proteins [Nishi, 2002; Sun-Wada, 2004; Smith, 2003; Faundez, 2004].

The v-ATPases are multi-subunit complexes that are composed of two domains. The V1 domain is a peripheral complex of 640 kDa that consists of eight different subunits (A–H) and is responsible for ATP hydrolysis. The V0 domain is an integral complex of 260 kDa, which includes five different subunits (a, d, c, c' and c'') and is responsible for proton translocation.

Table 2 shows the nomenclature, molecular mass and subunit function (if known) of the v-ATPase components [Nishi, 2002]. Structurally, the v-ATPases resemble the ATP synthases (or F-ATPases), which synthesise ATP in mitochondria, chloroplasts and bacteria. Since it has been established that F-ATPases exhibit rotational catalysis, a rotary mechanism has also been assumed for v-ATPases and is supported by recent studies [Nishi 2002, Sennoune 2004].

| Subunits of the v-ATPase | | | | | |
|---|---|---|---|---|---|
| Domain | Subunit | Iso-forms | Nomenclature | MW (kDa) | Proposed function/location |
| V1 (Peripheral stalk) | A | | ATP6V1A | 70 | Catalytic ATP-binding, regulation |
| | B | B1, B2 | ATPV1B(1,2) | 56 | Noncatalytic ATP-binding |
| | C | C1, C2 | ATPV1C(1,2) | 42 | Peripheral stator |
| | D | | ATPV1D | 34 | Central rotor |
| | E | E1, E2 | ATPV1E(1,2) | 31 | Peripheral stator |
| | F | | ATPV1F | 14 | Central rotor |
| | G | G1, G2, G3 | ATPV1G(1,2,3) | 13 | Peripheral stator |
| | H | | ATPV1H | 50 | Peripheral stator |
| V0 (Membrane sector) | A | a1-a4 | ATPV0A(1,2,4)/TCIRG1 | 100 | Peripheral stator, $H^+$ translocation |
| | D | d1-d2 | ATPV0D(1,2) | 38 | Non-integral membrane component |
| | C | | ATP6V0C | 16 | $H^+$ translocation |
| | c'' | | ATP6V0B | 21 | $H^+$ translocation |
| | E | | ATP6V0E | 9 | Membrane sector associated |

Table 2: Subunits of the v-ATPase [modified from Nishi, 2002; Smith, 2003]

### 1.2.3.2 Voltage-gated chloride channels (ClC-channels)

The activity of the v-ATPase is electrogenic, i.e. the accumulation of positively charged protons in organelles generates a transmembrane electric gradient. This inside-positive membrane potential constitutes a major factor in determining the degree of acidification, since it provides a force that opposes the activity of the proton pump. Hence, pathways of anion influx and cation efflux dissipate the membrane potential and regulate intravesicular pH. It is believed that inwardly directed chloride channels play an important role in the pH homeostasis of intracellular compartments, and recent discoveries revealed the important position of the ClC-family of chloride channels in this context (see Figure 1) [Faundez, 2004].

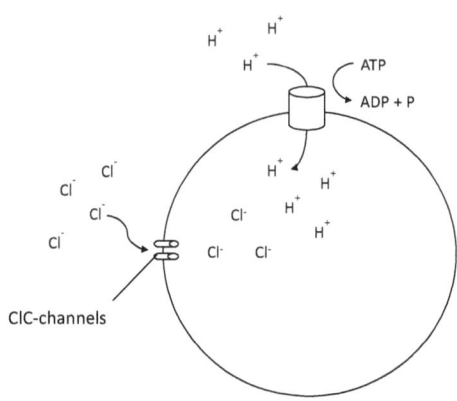

**Figure 1:** Role of ClC-channels in the regulation of vesicular acidification

Jentsch et al. discovered the ClC gene family in 1990 by cloning ClC-0, enriched in the electric organ of the marine ray Torpedo [Jentsch, 1990]. Today the ClC-channels constitute the largest known family of chloride channels. They can be found in organisms from prokaryotes to mammals, in which they comprise nine genes. ClC-1, ClC-2, ClC-Ka and ClC-Kb are expressed in the plasma membrane, while ClC-3 to ClC-7 localise predominantly to intracellular compartments [Faundez, 2004]. The latter can be divided into two branches according to their genetic homology: ClC-3 to ClC-5 share an 80% sequence identity, while ClC-6 and ClC-7 have 45% of their genetic sequence in common [Jentsch, Poët, et al., 2005].

ClC-proteins are ubiquitously expressed and involved in a broad variety of physiological processes. Plasma membrane ClC-channels play a role in the stabilization of membrane potential, cell volume regulation, transepithelial transport and extracellular acidification. Intracellular ClC-channels are involved in synaptic signalling, endocytic trafficking and vesicular acidification. Human genetic diseases due to mutations in ClC-channels likewise underline their physiological importance [Dutzler, 2007; Jentsch, Poët, et al., 2005]. Mutations of ClC-1, ClC-5 and ClC-7 were found to cause myotonia, Dent's disease, and osteopetrosis, respectively [Faundez, 2004].

Several studies point to a key role of ClC-3, -5 and -7 in endosomal and lysosomal acidification, with ClC-7 localising predominantly to the lysosomal compartment [Faundez, 2004; Jentsch, Neagoe, and Scheel, 2005; Dutzler, 2007; Hara-Chikuma, 2004; Kasper, 2005; Li, 2002].

All members of the ClC-family share a conserved molecular architecture. Their structural organization includes a complex transmembrane transport domain that is usually followed by a cytoplasmatic component. The latter is believed to play an important role in transport regulation [Dutzler, 2007]. ClC-channels function as homodimers in which each monomer has its own pore (double-barrelled channels). Each pore of the dimer (protopore) retains its individual properties, such as ion selectivity and single-channel conductance, and can be opened and closed by an individual gate independently of the state of the other gate. In addition to the protopore gate, there is also (at least in ClC-0 and ClC-1) a common gate that closes both pores in parallel [Jentsch, Poët, et al., 2005]. ClC-channels can be modulated by voltage, extra- and intracellular anions, pH, extracellular $Ca^{2+}$, cell swelling, and phosphorylation. The voltage-dependence is thought to result from the movement of the permanent anion, acting as a gating charge, within the protopore. This model renders gating dependent on both $Cl^-$-concentration and voltage [Jentsch, Poët, et al., 2005]. Although most of the ClC-channels function as gated anion channels, some of them might work as $H^+/Cl^-$-exchangers, a possibility which is especially discussed for ClC-3, ClC-4 and ClC-5 [Jentsch, Neagoe, and Scheel, 2005; Zifarelli, 2007].

Table 3 gives an overview of function and localisation of mammalian ClC chloride channels.

**Function and localisation of mammalian ClC-channels**

| Name | Tissue | Membrane | Function | Mouse model | Human disease |
|---|---|---|---|---|---|
| ClC-1 | Skeletal muscle | PM | Stabilization of membrane potential | Myotonia | Myotonia (recessive and dominant) |
| ClC-2 | Broad | PM (baso-lateral in intestine) | Epithelial transport, regulation of pH, cell volume regulation | Degeneration of testes and retina | Epilepsy? |
| ClC-Ka+ barttin | Kidney and ear | PM (baso-lateral) | Epithelial transport | Diabetes insipidus | |
| ClC-Kb+ barttin | | PM (baso-lateral) | Epithelial transport | | Barter III renal salt loss |
| ClC-3 | Broad | Endosomes, synaptic vesicles | Endosomal and/or synaptic vesicle acidification | CNS degeneration (loss of hippocampus, blindness) | |
| ClC-4 | Brain, muscle, liver | ER, SR, endosomes | Endosomal acidification? | | |
| ClC-5 | Kidney, intestine | Endosomes | Endosomal acidification, endocytosis | Proteinuria, change in calciotropic hormones | Dent's disease, proteinuria, kidney stones |
| ClC-6 | Broad | ER, endosomes | Endosomal acidification? | | |
| ClC-7 | Broad | Late endosomes, lysosomes | Lysosomal acidification/ resorption lacuna of osteoclasts | Osteopetrosis, blindness, lysosomal storage disease | Osteopetrosis (recessive and dominant) |

**Table 3:** Function and localisation of mammalian ClC-channels [modified from Jentsch, Poët, et al., 2005; Jentsch, Neagoe, and Scheel, 2005]

### 1.2.4 V-ATPase and ClC-channels in cancer and drug resistance

Several studies have investigated the role of the v-ATPase in drug resistance. Despite its major involvement in vesicular acidification, most attention has been paid to plasmalemmal expression of the v-ATPase. Residing in the plasma membrane of human cancer cells, it may participate in cell growth, differentiation, angiogenesis and metastasis. As extracellular acidity constitutes, for instance, an essential factor of invasiveness and proliferation, expression of v-ATPases may provide an acidic microenvironment and thus facilitate the development of metastatic disease [Sennoune, 2004, Torigoe, 2002, Izumi, 2003]. However, the 'ion-trapping hypothesis' suggests a link between compartmental acidification, provided by the v-ATPase, and resistance to weak-base chemotherapeutic drugs. Especially for the weak-base anthracyclines daunomycin and adriamycin, several studies showed that a disruption of lysosomal pH with concanamycin A in drug resistant cell lines could induce a nucleo-cytoplasmic redistribution of previously sequestered drugs and restore drug sensitivity [Ouar, 2003; Atlan, 1998; Moriyama, 1994; Raghunand, 2000].

Far less attention has been paid to a possible involvement of ClC-channels in drug resistance [Weylandt, Nebrig, 2007; Suh, 2005]. Recently, Olsen et al. suggested that voltage-gated chloride channels might be important for cell proliferation and invasive cell migration of primary brain tumours and derived cells. His group could show that ClC-2, -3, and -5 channels are expressed at high levels in biopsies from low- and high-grade malignant gliomas and that Cl⁻ currents are mediated by ClC-2 and ClC-3 in glioma cell lines. However, the study focused on plasma membrane expression of ClC-channels and discussed their potential role in rapid changes of cell size and shape during tissue invasion [Olsen, 2003]. First evidence for an involvement of intracellular ClC-channels in drug resistance was given by Weylandt, Nebrig et al. By transfecting the neuroendocrine tumour cell line BON with GFP-tagged ClC-3, it could be shown that ClC-3 localised to the lysosomal compartment, that BON cells over-expressing ClC-3 had more acidic compartments, and that these cells were more resistant to the weak-base cytotoxic drug etoposide than control cells [Weylandt, Nebrig 2007].

## 1.3 Etoposide

Etoposide was introduced in 1971 and is currently used for the treatment of small cell lung cancer, testicular cancer, lymphomas and metastatic high grade neuroendocrine tumours. Chemically, it is a weak base with a pKa of 9.8. As a derivative of podophyllotoxin it inhibits DNA synthesis by inducing double- and single-strand DNA breaks. This cytotoxic action is thought to be due to the interference of etoposide with the scission-reunion reaction of mammalian topoisomerase [Van Maanen, 1988; Meresse, 2004]. Because of its chemical properties and field of application, it constitutes a suitable drug to investigate the "protonation, sequestration and secretion model" in neuroendocrine tumour cells.

## 1.4 Aim of this study

Drug resistance constitutes a major challenge in the treatment of metastatic neuroendocrine cancer. Chemotherapeutic regimes for these tumours employ weak-base drugs such as, for instance, etoposide. Especially for this medication, a mechanism of resistance was suggested that linked increased acidification of intracellular compartments to the evolution of drug resistance. So far, most research groups have focused on the role of the driving force behind compartmental acidification, the vacuolar $H^+$-ATPase, in drug resistance. However, chloride channels of the ClC-family also play a pivotal role in the pH homeostasis of cellular organelles; Weylandt, Nebrig et al. provided first evidence that over-expression of ClC-3 could confer a drug resistant phenotype due to increased compartmental acidification. Following this finding, our work aims to further elucidate the role of ClC-channels and compartmental acidification in the evolution of etoposide resistance.

We addressed the problem through two different experimental approaches. On the one hand, we cultivated neuroendocrine tumour cells under long-term exposure to the v-ATPase inhibitor concanamycin A in order to select for increased ability to acidify intracellular compartments; then we assessed etoposide sensitivity as a function of altered pH homeostasis. On the other hand, we generated an etoposide-resistant neuroendocrine tumour cell line by exposing cells directly to etoposide, and then we examined compartmental acidity as a function of etoposide resistance. Our experiments included mapping vesicular acidity with a FACS assay, which had recently been established in our laboratory, as well as investigation of the gene expression of ClC-channels and the v-ATPase in qPCR. Since there are no adequate antibodies for the ClC-channels commercially available, it was one of our major aims to establish a reliable qPCR assay for these channels.

# 2 Materials and methods

## 2.1 Materials

Chemicals and reagents were purchased from Sigma-Aldrich, Invitrogen or Roche Applied Sciences. Tissue culture plastic ware was supplied by BD Biosciences (Falcon). Cell proliferation kit II and first strand cDNA synthesis kit were obtained from Roche Applied Sciences. RNA-Bee-RNA isolation reagent was purchased from AMS Biotechnology Ltd., QuantiTect SYBR Green PCR kit from Qiagen.

The FACS buffer contained PBS, 1% FBS and 25mM HEPES, and had a pH of 7.2 and an osmolarity of 295mosm.

## 2.2 Methods

### 2.2.1 Cell culture and generation of resistant cell lines

Lundqvist et al. established the LCC-18 cell line in 1986 from a poorly differentiated neuroendocrine colonic carcinoma of a 27-year-old patient. The patient showed clinical signs of a carcinoid syndrome, which included vomiting, diarrhoea and fever. Immunochemical investigation of the tumour showed positivity for neuroendocrine markers such as vasoactive intestinal polypeptide (VIP), synaptophysin, tyrosine hydroxylase and L-dopa decarboxylase. In the culture medium high concentrations of VIP and glucagon could be found and the cells retained their endocrine characteristics through more than 100 passages [Lundqvist, 1991]. Accordingly, LCC-18 constitutes a suitable model in order to investigate gastrointestinal neuroendocrine tumours.

LCC-18 cells were grown at 37°C in a 5% $CO_2$, water-saturated incubator. The culture medium included RPMI-1640, 10% FBS, 0.5% ITS liquid media supplement and 10μg/ml ciprofloxacin. Medium was exchanged every 1-3 days and passages 45-65 were used in all experiments.

Resistant cell lines were obtained by treating the cells with initially high doses of etoposide (up to 5μM) or concanamycin A (up to 10nM). Since the cells could not survive at such high drug concentrations, doses were successively lowered over a period of 3 weeks until an endpoint of permanent culture in 1μM etoposide or 1nM concanamycin A was achieved. Experiments for both drug-selected and control cells were performed in drug-free medium.

### 2.2.2 Quantification of acridine orange fluorescence from acidic compartments

Acridine orange (AO) is a fluorescent, weakly basic amine. While it is cell membrane permeable in unprotonated state, it accumulates in acidic compartments of cells where it is trapped due to protonation. When concentrations of AO rise, the spontaneous formation of oligomeric AO molecules leads to a shift in fluorescence emission maxima from green (526nm band) to far red (680nm band), and acidic compartments are, thus, labelled in red [Millot, 1997]. The accumulation in acidic compartments depends on the extracellular AO concentration and is proportional to the magnitude of the pH gradient across the compartmental membrane; or if more than one membrane separates the intracellular from the external compartment, it is dependent on the overall net pH gradient. Moreover, when the external pH is kept constant, the compartmental AO concentration is linearly proportional to the external AO concentration and the slope of their interdependence represents the pH gradient. Since fluorescence emission intensity depends also linearly on the AO concentration, the acidity of intracellular compartments can be reliably assessed by exposing cell populations to several external AO concentrations at a constant external pH, measuring the corresponding AO emission intensities in far red, plotting them against the external AO concentrations and determining the slopes of their interdependence [Ursos, 2000; Weylandt, Nebrig, et al. 2007].

LCC-18 cells were washed with PBS, detached from the culture flasks by trypsinization and re-suspended in FACS buffer. In preliminary experiments, an AO concentration range from 0.1µM to 5µM with an incubation time of 8 minutes was found to suffice for reaching a steady state of AO accumulation. Accordingly, samples with AO concentrations from 0.25µM – 2µM were prepared and cells were incubated for 8 minutes at room temperature. Fluorescence emission was then examined by flow cytometry (FACScan, BD Biosciences). For each external AO concentration 10,000 cells were assessed. Cells were excited with the 488nm argon-ion laser and the emitted fluorescence intensity was measured in the FL-3 channel (> 670nm Low-pass filter). The mean FL-3 intensity values were plotted against the external AO concentration and fitted with a linear regression of the first order with the Marquardt-Levenberg algorithm based on the least square method (SigmaPlot, version

2001). The slopes were validated statistically by F-test of parallelism (R Development Core Team (2008); R: A language and environment for statistical computing; R Foundation for Statistical Computing, Vienna, Austria; http://www.R-project.org). Based on analysis of covariance (ANCOVA), the test answers the question whether a model with lines of different slopes provides a significant better fit of the data than a model with parallel lines. Statistical relevance was assumed for $p < 0.05$, and at least 3 independent measurements were performed for each treatment.

### 2.2.3 Cell proliferation assay

Drug cytotoxicity was investigated using the cell proliferation kit II (Roche). The assay is based on the reduction of the yellow tetrazolium salt XTT. In vital cells, XTT is converted by mitochondrial dehydrogenases into an orange, water-soluble dye whose concentration can be evaluated by measuring absorption at 450-500 nm.

Cells, cultured as described above, were washed twice with 10ml PBS, detached with 2ml trypsin and re-suspended in 10ml culture medium without phenol red (in order to avoid interference with the absorption readings). Cells were counted in a haemocytometer and diluted with culture medium until a concentration of 250 cells/µl was achieved. In order to investigate optimal seeding density, growth curves were performed. We considered that an optimal seeding density was achieved when cells grew in the linear range of the growth curve without any signs of cell death by overgrowth after 3 days in culture. Furthermore, the growth curves enabled us to exclude changes in growth properties due to the generation of resistant cell lines. 25,000 cells/well were seeded in 96-well tissue culture plates and cultured in an incubator at 37°C, 5% $CO_2$ water vapour-saturated atmosphere. After 24 hours the culture medium was replaced by fresh medium containing different concentrations of etoposide (stock solution in DMSO). Cells were cultured in the presence of the drug for another 48 hours before the cell viability was assessed. 5ml XTT reagent was thawed and mixed with 0.1ml of the electron coupling reagent PMS (N-methyl-dibenzopyrazine methyl sulfate). 50µl of the solution was added to each well. After 18 hours, incubation plates were read in an ELISA reader at 450nm and at 650nm as control for background absorption.

The percentage of cell survival was expressed as normalized average absorption values from 4 replicates per each drug concentration ± standard error. Concentration response curves were obtained by fitting the experimental data by non-linear regression with a logistic curve (SigmaPlot, version 2001). The concentration of drug required to decrease cell proliferation by 50% ($IC_{50}$) was determined for each treatment from the concentration response curve of the XTT assay and statistically compared by Student's t-test. Statistical relevance was assumed for $p < 0.05$. Two and three independent measurements were performed for etoposide-resistant and concanamycin A-resistant cells, respectively.

## 2.2.4 Quantitative real time polymerase chain reaction (qPCR)

### 2.2.4.1 General considerations

Quantitative real time PCR allows a relative quantification of gene expression in biological samples by measuring the amount of specific mRNA. There are different methodological approaches to qPCR and we employed an assay based on the DNA-binding fluorescent dye Sybr Green. In brief, our approach included the following three independent steps: First, RNA of the biological sample was isolated. It was then transcribed into complementary DNA (cDNA) with the help of a reverse transcriptase (RT reaction). Thirdly, a specific sequence of the cDNA was amplified by means of a thermostable DNA-dependent DNA polymerase. Specificity was achieved by careful selection of primers. The final assay contained the fluorescent dye whose signal was proportional to the amount of DNA in the sample, and allowed us to deduce the quantity of original mRNA. As Sybr Green, a very sensitive, double-stranded DNA (dsDNA) binding dye, attaches to any dsDNA, a careful design of primers and thorough validation of the qPCR results are necessary in order to obtain reliable results [Bustin, 2004; Bustin, 2000].

### 2.2.4.2 Isolation of RNA

Isolation of RNA was performed with the RNA-Bee-RNA isolation procedure. RNA-Bee is a monophase solution, which operates on the basis of phenol and quanidine thiocyanate. Cells, cul-tured as mentioned above, were grown in $75cm^2$ culture dishes to approximately 70% confluence, washed twice with 10ml PBS and lysed directly in the culture dish by addition of 1ml RNA-Bee. The lysate was collected with cell scratchers and transferred into a 1.5ml Eppendorf tube. 200μl chloroform was added, tubes were vigorously shaken for 30 seconds, stored on ice for 5 minutes and centrifuged for 15 minutes at 12,000g in a table-centrifuge. The upper, aqueous phase containing RNA was carefully transferred into a new tube, while DNA and proteins remained in a lower, organic phase. Pure RNA was obtained from the aqueous phase by precipitating it with 0.5ml isopropanol, storing it for 10 minutes at room temperature and subsequently centrifuging it. The RNA pellet was washed twice with 1ml 75% ethanol and solubilised in distilled ribonuclease free water. Depending on the size of the RNA pellet, 50μl to 250μl water was added.

In order to determine the RNA content, the optical density was measured at 260nm ($OD_{260}$) in a NanoDrop 1000 (Thermo Fisher Scientific) and the RNA concentration was calculated using the following formula: RNA concentration = $OD_{260}$ * dilution factor * (40μg RNA/1000μl) [μg/μl]. Different amounts of ribonuclease-free water were added and measurements repeated until concentrations of approximately 1μg RNA/μl were achieved.

### 2.2.4.3 Reverse transcription (RT)

2μg of total RNA per sample was used in RT reaction with the first strand cDNA synthesis kit (Roche). The following table shows the reaction mix:

| Reaction mixture for RT reaction | |
|---|---|
| Reagents | Volume |
| 10x Reaction buffer | 2μl |
| 25mM $MgCl_2$ | 4μl |
| Deoxynucleotide mix | 2μl |
| Random primer p(dN)$_6$ | 2μl |
| RNAse inhibitor | 1μl |
| AMV enzyme | 0.8μl |
| RNA sample | 2 μg |
| Sterile water | Add to 20μl |
| Total | 20μl |

**Table 4:** Reaction mixture for RT reaction

The reaction was performed by incubation for 1 hour in a 42°C water bath. Finally, 180μl of distilled water was added in order to achieve a final concentration equivalent to 10ng RNA/μl.

## 2.2.4.4 Primer design

The RT reaction reverse transcribes every type of RNA in the sample. Hence, we had to assume that not only cDNA of the mRNA of our target genes, but also cDNA of other RNA was present in the sample. Moreover, contamination of the sample with original DNA could not be excluded. Therefore, the primer sequence for a particular gene had to be both specific for the gene and only present in the cDNA of the corresponding mRNA, i.e. it should not be found in the original DNA or in cDNA of other RNA than the target mRNA. This demand could be addressed by ensuring that primers were located in the transcript at an exon-exon boundary and spanned at least one intron [Bustin, 2004; Bustin, 2000].

The internet provides useful tools for primer design. A short summary of our procedure can be found in Table 5. First, reference sequences were searched in the nucleotide function of PubMed. The suggested sequences could then be used to find potential primers in PrimerBank. In order to ensure location at exon-exon boundaries, the transcript information was mapped with the Ensemble genome browser and the position of the primers in the transcript was validated.

**Procedure for primer design**

| Step | Search for | Website | Procedure |
|---|---|---|---|
| 1 | Reference sequence | NCBI - PubMed http://www.ncbi.nlm.nih.gov/sites/entrez?db=PubMed | "Nucleotide" mode; reference sequence by name of gene/protein of interest |
| 2 | Primer | PrimerBank http://pga.mgh.harvard.edu/primerbank/ | Primers by reference sequence |
| 3 | Location in transcript | Ensemble genome browser http://www.ensembl.org/index.html | Transcript information by reference sequence; localisation of primer in transcript sequence; exon-exon boundary? Introns spanned? |

**Table 5:** Procedure for primer design

The following table shows the such-designed primers for our experiments.

## Sequences of qPCR primers

| Gene | | Primer Sequence 5' → 3' | Annealing temp. [°C] | Amplicon size (bp) |
|---|---|---|---|---|
| ABCB1 | Sense | TGGTTCAGGTGGCTCTGGAT | 60 | 71 |
| | Antisense | CTGTAGACAAACGATGAGCTATCACA | 60 | |
| ABCB4 | Sense | ACCGACTGTCTACGGTCCGAA | 60 | 295 |
| | Antisense | TCCATCGGTTTCCACATCAAGG | 60 | |
| ABCC1 | Sense | CAATGCTGTGATGGCGATG | 60 | 65 |
| | Antisense | GATCCGATTGTCTTTGCTCTTCA | 60 | |
| ABCC3 | Sense | ATTTGGAATCTAACATCGTGGCT | 60 | 153 |
| | Antisense | GCCGGTAGCGCACAGAATA | 62.2 | |
| ATPV1A | Sense | GGACCTGTGGTTACAGCCTG | 62.2 | 123 |
| | Antisense | CACCTGAATAGTAGCCATGTCAC | 60.4 | |
| CLC-3 | Sense | GAGAGGGATAAATGTCCACAGTG | 60 | 114 |
| | Antisense | ACTCAAGGCCCAGAAGATGTA | 60 | |
| CLC-5 | Sense | GAGGAGCCAATCCCTGGTGTA | 63 | 101 |
| | Antisense | TTGGTAATCTCTCGGTGCCTA | 60 | |
| CLC-7 | Sense | TCTGCGCTTTTCCGAGTCG | 62.6 | 75 |
| | Antisense | AGGGTCCATATCCGGGTCC | 62.2 | |
| HPRT1 | Sense | CCTGGCGTCGTGATTAGTGAT | 61.9 | 131 |
| | Antisense | AGACGTTCAGTCCTGTCCATAA | 60.5 | |
| P21 | Sense | CCTGTCACTGTCTTGTACCCT | 60 | 130 |
| | Antisense | GCGTTTGGAGTGGTAGAAATCT | 60 | |
| RPLPO | Sense | GGCGACCTGGAAGTCCAACT | 60 | 149 |
| | Antisense | CCATCAGCACCACAGCCTTC | 60 | |
| TBP | Sense | TGCACAGGAGCCAAGAGTGAA | 60 | 132 |
| | Antisense | CACATCACAGCTCCCCACCA | 60 | |
| 18S rRNA | Sense | CGGCTACCACATCCAAGGAA | 60 | 186 |
| | Antisense | GCTGGAATTACCGCGGCT | 60 | |

**Table 6:** Sequences of qPCR primers (ABCB1 to C3: Adenosine triphosphate binding cassette transporter B1 to C3; ATPV1A: Vacuolar (proton) adenosine triphosphatase, domain V1, subunit A; HPRT1: Hypoxanthine phosphoribosyltransferase 1; RPLPO: Large ribosomal protein P0; TBP: TATA-binding protein)

### 2.2.4.5 Quantitative polymerase chain reaction

qPCR was performed using the QuantiTect SYBR Green RT-PCR kit (Qiagen). Sample preparation was realised under a PCR-hood in order to avoid contamination. First a master mix with DNA polymerase was prepared and distributed to tubes that contained a sufficient amount of sample for duplicates. Finally, the samples were transferred to 96 well plates. Each well contained a sample equivalent to 50ng of original RNA before RT reaction in the following mixture:

| Reaction mixture for qPCR | |
|---|---|
| Reagents | Volume |
| SensiMix | 11.25 µl |
| 50x Sybr Green | 0.45 µl |
| 100µM Sense primer | 0.1125 µl |
| 100µM Antisense primer | 0.1125 µl |
| Sterile water | 5.575 µl |
| Sample [10ng RNA/µl] | 5 µl |
| Total | 22.5 µl |

**Table 7:** Reaction mixture for qPCR

The plate was centrifuged for 1 minute at 1000g in order to ensure that the samples were located at the bottom of the wells. Then, qPCR was carried out with a DNA engine Opticon 2 continuous fluorescence detector (Bio-Rad). The QuantiTect SYBR Green RT-PCR master mix contains HotStarTaq DNA polymerase, which requires initial thermal activation. Cycling conditions can be seen in table 8. Finally a melting curve was created in order to control the specificity of the amplification.

| Cycling conditions for qPCR | | |
|---|---|---|
| Step | Temperature | Time/Procedure |
| Enzyme activation | 95 °C | 10 minutes |
| Denaturation | 95 °C | 15 seconds |
| Annealing | 60 °C | 30 seconds |
| Extension | 72 °C | 15 seconds |
| Data acquisition | (72 °C) | Read plate |
| Cycles (2-40) | - | Continue 39 more times to line 2 |
| Melting curve | 60 – 95 C | Hold 1 second at each 1°C and read |

**Table 8:** Cycling conditions for qPCR

### *2.2.4.6 Analysis*

The assessment of every gene of a plate included two negative controls and a standard curve. The negative controls consisted of one duplicate of distilled water and one duplicate of reaction mix without a biologic sample. In order to create a standard curve, one sample was measured at five different dilutions.

As the initial step of analysis, the melting curve was evaluated. Since every amplification product had a specific temperature of denaturation, the melting curve allowed a control of the specificity of the reaction. Thus, formation of primer dimers or co-amplification of other genetic sequences could be excluded.

The data obtained by the Opticon cycler described the fluorescence intensity of a sample in relation to the number of cycles. At a particular cycle number the emission of every sample showed an exponential growth and rose above background noise. For every gene of a plate we set manually a threshold line and determined for every sample the number of cycles to reach that line (Ct value). The Ct value is inversely proportional to the logarithm of the initial amount of mRNA template in the sample. Every Ct value could thus be related to the original quantity of mRNA by means of linear standard curves. Finally, duplicates were averaged and normalised to the control cell line and to internal reference genes (see below).

### *2.2.4.7 Statistic analysis*

Every experiment was performed three times. Cells were split and grown in separate flasks under identical conditions. RNA isolation, RT reaction and qPCR were then realised simultaneously, and qPCR was performed on the same plate. Thus we could assume that we compared two different groups, e.g. 1µM etoposide-resistant cells and control cells, in our experiments, each in three replicates. A non-paired t-test was applied for statistical analysis and standard errors were calculated between the replicates. The gene expression is shown as an average of these replicates, and statistical relevance was assumed for $p < 0.05$.

# 3 Results

## 3.1 LCC-18 Resistant to 1nM concanamycin A

### 3.1.1 Generation and vesicular acidity of LCC-18 resistant to 1nM concanamycin A

In order to investigate intracellular acidity as a factor in drug resistance, we decided to select a cell line by long-term exposure to concanamycin A. Concanamycin A is a specific inhibitor of the vesicular proton pump. It binds to the subunit c of its stalk and thus inhibits its rotational action and, consequently, vesicular acidification [Bowman, 2004]. We hypothesized that impaired acidification might be sensed by homeostatic cellular mechanisms and result in an up-regulation of vesicle acidification mechanisms such as intracellular ClC-channels. As a result, vesicular acidity and etoposide resistance might be increased.

A stable LCC-18 cell line resistant to 1nM concanamycin A was established as described above. Subsequently, vesicular acidity was evaluated by the acridine orange-based FACS assay, which was previously established in our laboratory (see Materials and Methods). As described above in detail, the assay allows an estimation of the acidity of intracellular organelles by comparing the slopes of regression lines of the interdependence of fluorescence intensity and external AO concentration. As shown in figure 2 the slope of such a regression line for 1nM concanamycin A-resistant cells was significantly higher than that for control cells, with 90 versus 74 ($R^2 > 0.99$, $p < 0.001$, F-test of parallelism), respectively. Organelles could thus be considered more acidic.

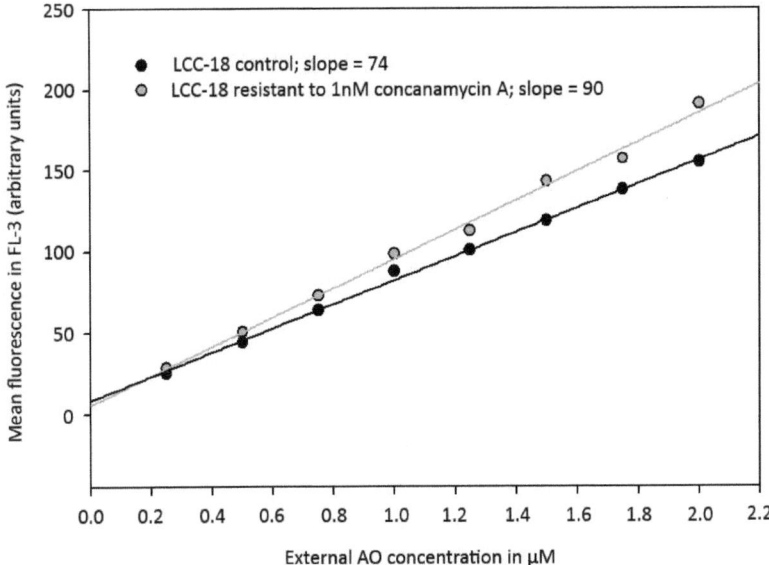

**Figure 2:** FACS assay of LCC-18 resistant to 1nM concanamycin A in comparison to control cells. Each point represents 10,000 cells. Experimental values were fitted with linear regression lines of the first order (SigmaPlot, version 2001; $R^2 > 0.99$) and compared by F-test of parallelism. The slopes of the regression lines are significantly different ($p < 0.001$).

## 3.1.2 Etoposide sensitivity of LCC-18 resistant to 1nM concanamycin A

Subsequently, we analysed whether etoposide sensitivity was altered in the course of the selection process, potentially due to increased vesicular acidity. Therefore, concanamycin A-selected cells were examined in a colorimetric cell proliferation assay based on XTT (see Materials and Methods) and exposed to different concentrations of etoposide. As shown in Figure 3 the concanamycin A-selected cells were more resistant to etoposide than control cells with an $IC_{50}$ of 493µM ± 10µM in comparison to 48µM ± 1µM ($R^2 > 0.99$, $p < 0.001$, Student's t-test).

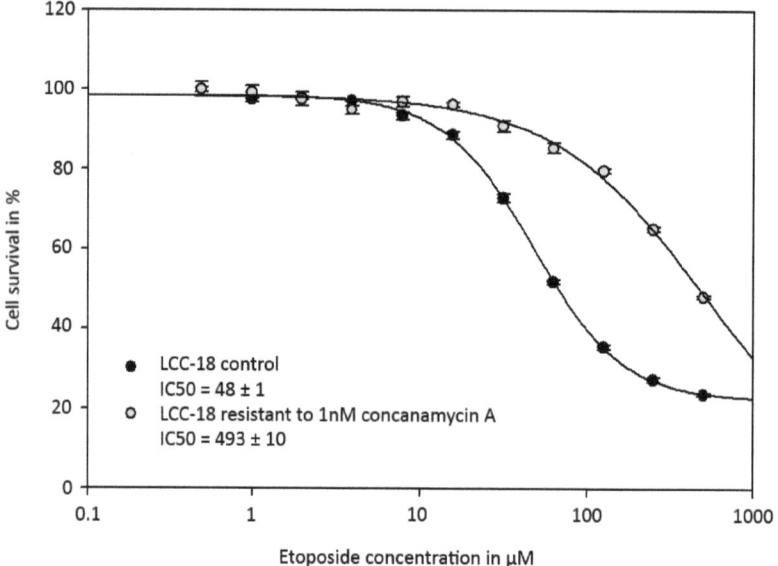

**Figure 3:** Cell proliferation assay of LCC-18 resistant to 1nM concanamycin A in comparison to control cells. 25,000 cells/well were seeded on a 96 well plate in quadruplicates. The averaged experimental data were fitted by non-linear regression with a logistic curve (SigmaPlot, version 2001; $R^2 > 0.99$). The $IC_{50}$s of the two tested cell populations were significantly different ($p < 0.001$, Student's t-test).

## 3.1.3 Genetic expression of LCC-18 resistant to 1nM concanamycin A

In order to gain a more complete understanding of the processes responsible for increased vesicular acidification and etoposide resistance in the concanamycin A-selected LCC-18 cell line, the genetic expression of potentially involved proteins was examined. As mentioned above, a multidrug-resistant phenotype is often associated with an overexpression of members of the ATP-binding cassette family of proteins (ABC transporters). Moreover, etoposide has been characterised as a substrate of ABCB1, C1 and C3, also named Pgp, MRP1 and MRP3, respectively [Ambudkar, 1999; Borst, 2000; Zelcer, 2001]. Accordingly, we decided to include two major groups in our investigation: on the one hand the ABC transporters ABCC1, C3, B1 and, additionally, B4. On the other hand, proteins with a key role in vesicular acidification were tested: here we chose the vesicular $H^+$-ATPase (subunit A), the main driving force of vesicular acidification, and ClC-3, -5 and -7 as members of the ClC-family of chloride channels implicated in the regulation of the vesicular pH. Ideally, an exploration of protein expression would be realized by direct assessment of protein levels. Unfortunately, there are no specific antibodies commercially available for the ClC-channels. This is why we decided to focus our investigation on mRNA expression using a quantitative PCR approach.

### *3.1.3.1 Establishment of the real time PCR assay*

Although real time PCR is a powerful and frequently used technique for quantifying mRNA expression in biological samples, a number of problems are associated with its use. These include the inherent variability of RNA in biological samples, variability of extraction protocols that may co-purify inhibitors, and different reverse transcription and PCR efficiencies. Consequently, it is important that primers are designed very carefully and that an accurate method of normalisation is chosen to control for errors [Bustin, 2004; Huggett, 2005].

### *3.1.3.1.1 Normalisation of qPCR data*

There are several procedures, which can easily be included into the qPCR protocol in order to minimize experimental error. We thus sought to achieve similar sample sizes, and we determined the RNA content by $OD_{260}$ to assure similar RNA quantities in the RT reaction (see Materials and Methods). The most common technique for normalisation is based on internal control genes, also referred to as housekeeping genes. A gene is considered a perfect housekeeper if it is expressed constantly in every sample, independently of its treatment. However, it has been shown that even very commonly used reference genes can exhibit a high variation of expression. Thus it is of use to explore several reference genes in order to search for those with the most stable expression profile and to normalize the data not only to one, but to several reference genes [Bustin, 2004].

In order to validate our internal control genes, we used a method recently proposed and developed by Vandesompele et al. using a program based on an excel platform called geNorm. GeNorm allows users to determine both the most stably expressed internal control genes out of a set of data and the number of housekeeper genes required for appropriate normalisation. Subsequently, a normalisation factor is calculated by geometric averaging [Vandesompele, 2002].

GeNorm relies on the assumption that if an internal control gene is expressed identically in every sample, the ratio of the expression of two of such genes must be constant. Thus for every potential control gene the program calculates the pairwise variation with all other control genes (as the standard deviation of the logarithmically transformed expression ratios) in a set of data. The average of that variation for a particular gene is defined as the stability measure (M-value) of the gene; in other words, the internal control genes can be ranked by their stability. In our investigation we included four housekeeping genes that were stably expressed in preliminary induction experiments. We made sure to select genes that belong to different functional classes in order to reduce the risk of co-regulation. Table 9 shows the four housekeeping genes including physiological function and M-values for concanamycin A and etoposide-resistant cells. TATA-binding protein (TBP), large ribosomal protein P0 (RPLPO) and hypoxanthine phosphoribosyltransferase 1 (HPRT1) in the concanamycin A-selected cell line, and TBP, HPRT1 and 18S rRNA in the etoposide-resistant cell line were found to be most stably expressed.

**M-value and physiological function of control genes**

| Control Gene | Physiological Function | M-value for concanamycin A-resistant cells | M-value for etoposide-resistant cells |
|---|---|---|---|
| HPRT 1 | Purine recycling | 0.539 | 0.283 |
| RPLPO | Protein synthesis | 0.406 | 0.347 |
| TBP | RNA polymerase II transcription factor | 0.406 | 0.255 |
| 18S rRNA | Protein synthesis | 0.672 | 0.312 |

**Table 9:** M-value and physiological function of control genes (HPRT1: Hypoxanthine phosphoribosyltransferase 1; RPLPO: Large ribosomal protein P0; TBP: TATA-binding protein)

In a second step, geNorm makes it possible to determine the number of housekeeping genes required for optimal normalisation. Based on geometric averaging, several normalisation factors are calculated by starting with the two best performing control genes and successively including the next most stably expressed genes. Finally, the pairwise variation of the sequential normalisation factors is calculated, and the optimal number of control genes is achieved when there is no significant variation between two sequential normalisation factors. Based on their data, Vandesompele et al. suggested a cut-off variation value of 0.15, below which the inclusion of an additional control gene is not required. The variations between normalisation factors based on two and three reference genes accounted for 0.126 for concanamycin A and 0.079 for etoposide-resistant cells. Thus we decided to normalize our data to the geometric mean of the above-mentioned three most stably expressed housekeeping genes for each cell line.

### 3.1.3.2 mRNA expression in LCC-18 resistant to 1nM concanamycin A

Figure 4 shows the mRNA expression of the investigated genes in the concanamycin A-selected cell line. Significant up-regulation was observed for ClC-3 by 2.13 ± 0.56 (p = 0.016) and ClC-7 by 1.76 ± 0.25 (p = 0.008). Neither the expression of the ABC transporters nor that of ATP6V1A, ClC-5 or p21 were significantly changed.

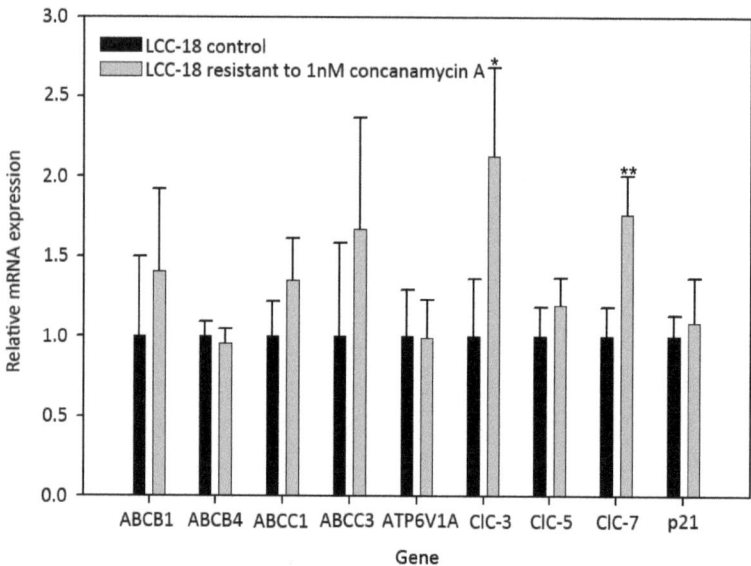

**Figure 4:** Gene expression of LCC-18 resistant to 1nM concanamycin A in relation to control cells. Values represent averages of three independent experiments, normalized to a factor based on the geometric average of TBP, HPRT1 and 18S rRNA (geNorm). Error bars indicate standard errors calculated between the three independent experiments, each of which was realised in duplicates. P-values accounted for p = 0.35 for ABCB1, p = 0.66 for ABCB4, p = 0.19 for ABCC1, p = 0.19 for ABCC3, p = 0.97 for ATP6V1A, p = 0.016 for ClC-3, p = 0.26 for ClC-5, p = 0.008 for ClC-7 and p = 0.76 for p21 (non-paired t-test, SigmaPlot 2001). Statistical significance was assumed for p < 0.05 (* indicates p < 0.05, ** p < 0.01).

## 3.2 LCC-18 resistant to 1μM etoposide

### 3.2.1 Generation of LCC-18 resistant to 1μM etoposide

While we investigated the pathway from experimentally altered pH homeostasis to etoposide resistance in the concanamycin A-selected cell line, we addressed the inverse pathway, i.e. from etoposide exposure to cellular pH homeostasis, in a second approach. Thus, we established a stable LCC-18 cell line resistant to 1μM etoposide as described above. In order to objectify the altered drug sensitivity, the XTT-based cell proliferation assay was performed (see Materials and Methods). As shown in Figure 5, the $IC_{50}$ of the resistant cell line was significantly higher than in control cells with 179μM ± 17μM versus 60μM ± 2μM ($R^2 > 0.99$, $p < 0.001$, Student's t-test). The assay thus demonstrated the enhanced drug resistance of the etoposide-selected cell line.

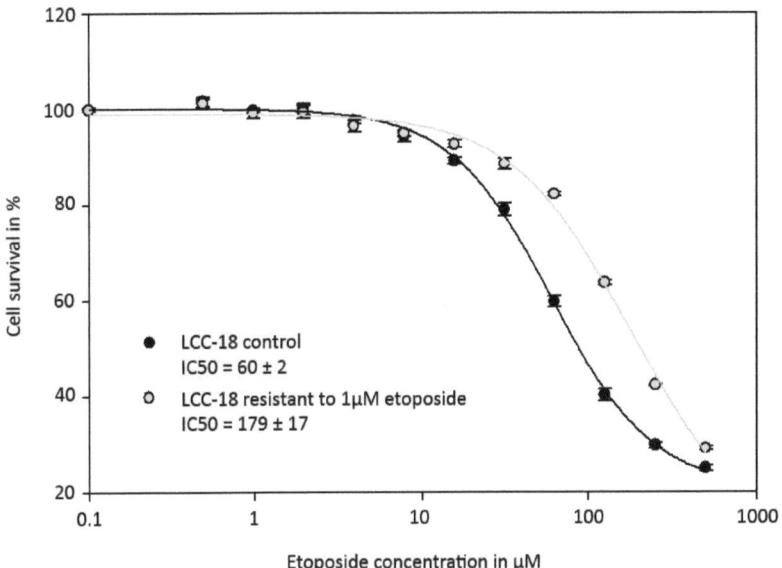

**Figure 5:** Cell proliferation assay of LCC-18 resistant to 1μM etoposide in comparison to control cells. 25,000 cells/well were seeded on a 96 well plate in quadruplicates. The averaged experimental data were fitted by non-linear regression with a logistic curve (SigmaPlot, version 2001, $R^2 > 0.99$). The $IC_{50}$s of the two tested cell populations were significantly different ($p < 0.001$, Student's t test).

## 3.2.2 Vesicular acidity of LCC-18 resistant to 1μM etoposide

In a second step we wanted to examine whether cellular pH homeostasis was changed in the course of the selection process. For this purpose, the etoposide-resistant cells were characterised using the AO-based FACS assay. Figure 6 shows the assessment of compartmental acidity in the etoposide-resistant cells in comparison to control cells. The regression line of selected cells showed a steeper slope than control cells with 105 versus 75 ($R^2 > 0.99$, $p < 0.001$, F-test of parallelism), respectively. Consequently, the intracellular organelles were more acidic in the etoposide-resistant cells than in control cells.

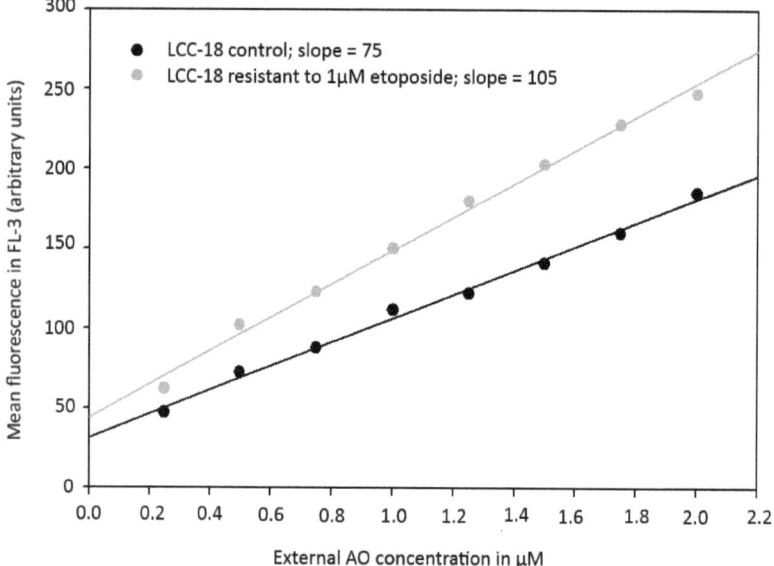

**Figure 6:** FACS assay of LCC-18 resistant to 1μM etoposide in comparison to control cells. Each point represents 10,000 cells. Experimental values were fitted with linear regression lines of the first order (SigmaPlot, version 2001, $R^2 > 0.99$) and compared by F-test of parallelism. The slopes of the regression lines are significantly different ($p < 0.001$).

### 3.2.3 mRNA expression in LCC-18 resistant to 1µM etoposide

In order to understand changes in genetic expression responsible for the altered phenotype of the 1µM etoposide-resistant cell line, we then investigated the target genes introduced above by means of the real time PCR assay. Figure 8 shows the relative expression of these genes of interest in the etoposide-resistant cell line normalised to control. P21 was included as a negative control as it is a very sensitive marker of apoptosis and was up-regulated up to 30-fold in preliminary experiments following treatment of LCC-18 cells with high doses of etoposide and concanamycin A. We assumed that unaltered expression of p21 in the resistant cell line would be a marker of stable growth. Its high average value shown in Figure 7 was due to up-regulation in one of the etoposide-resistant samples. However, since it remained normal in the other two samples, no statistical relevance could be found ($p = 0.2$).

Significant changes of mRNA expression could be observed for the drug efflux pumps ABCB4, ABCC1 and ABCC3, which were up-regulated by the factors $2.41 \pm 0.15$, $1.62 \pm 0.14$ and $1.59 \pm 0.15$, respectively. However, we did not observe any significant up-regulation of ABCB1, ATP6V1A, ClC-3, ClC-5 or ClC-7.

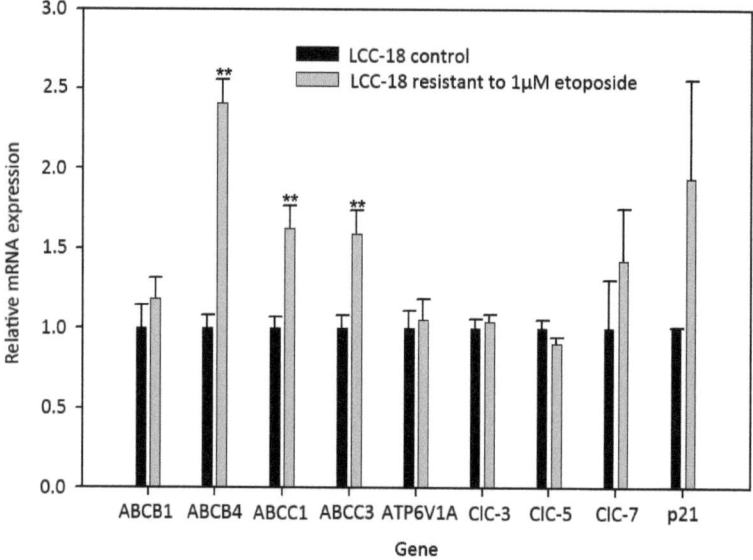

**Figure 7:** Gene expression of LCC-18 resistant to 1µM etoposide in relation to control cells. Values represent averages of three independent experiments, normalized to a factor based on the geometric average of TBP, HPRT1 and RPLPO (geNorm). Error bars indicate standard errors calculated between the three independent experiments, each of which was realised in duplicates. P-values accounted for $p = 0.2$ for ABCB1, $p < 0.0001$ for ABCB4, $p = 0.008$ for ABCC1, $p = 0.009$ for ABCC3, $p = 0.71$ for ATP6V1A, $p = 0.43$ for ClC-3, $p = 0.1$ for ClC-5, $p = 0.16$ for ClC-7 and $p = 0.2$ for p21 (non-paired t-test, SigmaPlot 2001). Statistical significance was assumed for $p < 0.05$ (* indicates $p < 0.05$, ** $p < 0.01$).

# 4 Discussion

## 4.1 LCC-18 resistant to 1nM concanamycin A

### 4.1.1 Vesicular acidity and etoposide resistance

This study aimed at understanding the relationship between vesicular acidity and etoposide resistance in a neuroendocrine tumor cell line. To achieve this, the LCC-18 cell line was first selected for an increased acidification phenotype by long-term exposure to concanamycin A. The plecomacrolide concanamycin A is an inhibitor of the subunit c of the vacuolar $H^+$-ATPase. We hypothesised that cells might overcome concanamycin A exposure by up-regulating vesicular acidification mechanisms, and as a result exhibit more acidic vesicles than parental cells. According to the 'protonation, sequestration and secretion model', enhanced compartmental acidification could exert a protective effect on cells against weak-base chemotherapeutic drugs like etoposide by trapping these drugs in acidic vesicles (see also Introduction). We hypothesised that this altered pH homeostasis of concanamycin A-selected cells might lead to enhanced etoposide resistance due to drug sequestration. Indeed LCC-18 cells selected for tolerance to 1nM concanamycin A had more acidic vesicles than control cells and were also more resistant to etoposide. This data supports the proposed link between compartmental acidity and etoposide resistance.

### 4.1.2 Gene expression, vesicular acidity and etoposide resistance

However, the experiments described could not exclude other mechanisms of cellular detoxification independent of intravesicular acidification. Particularly important in this context are the ABC transporters, which cover a very broad spectrum of xenobiotics [Szakács, 2006]. Concanamycin A could be a substrate of at least one of the ABC transporters, similar to macrolide antibiotics, which have been described as substrates of ABC transporters in bacteria [Jacquet, 2008].

To test for this alternative model - explaining concanamycin A resistance as a result of up-regulation of ABC transporters that would simultaneously protect against etoposide - an analysis of the expression of ABC transporters was included in the next experiment.

### 4.1.2.1 General considerations

Gene expression was analysed by qPCR. As we sought to elucidate how the compartmental pH decreased, we focused on mechanisms of pH regulation that included intracellular ClC-channels and the v-ATPase. Additionally, as mentioned above, we explored the extent to which an increased ABC transporter expression could account for decreased etoposide sensitivity.

While qPCR is a very powerful instrument to measure mRNA expression, the latter cannot directly be translated into protein expression. It has become increasingly clear that gene expression underlies considerable regulation at every step from DNA to protein. Translation depends, for instance, on cytoplasmic localisation of mRNA and mRNA packaging and storage, and includes control mechanisms such as micro RNAs (miRNAs) and short interfering RNAs (siRNAs) [Moore, 2005; Czaplinski, 2006; Rougemaille, 2008; Valencia-Sanchez, 2006; Shyu, 2008]. Hence, up-regulated mRNA expression points to but does not prove enhanced protein expression, and our data must be considered accordingly. This approach was chosen, however, as specific antibodies to several of the examined proteins (particularly the ClC-proteins) were not available, making the direct measurement of protein levels impossible.

### 4.1.2.2 Gene expression of concanamycin A-selected cells

In the concanamycin A-selected cell line, up-regulation of ClC-3 and ClC-7 was observed. Although ClC-7 expression was only 1.7-fold and ClC-3 expression 2.2-fold increased, these results can be considered reliable and relevant due to careful selection and validation of control genes. Both ClC-3 and ClC-7 can be localised to the endosomal compartment and are probably involved in vesicular acidification. Though ubiquitously expressed, ClC-3 resides predominantly in the nervous system and is associated with counter-ion currents for acidification of both synaptic vesicles and the late endosomal compartment [Jentsch, 2002]. As the cell line LCC-18 shows a high protein expression of ClC-3 [Weylandt, Nebrig, et al., 2007], and as up-regulation of ClC-3 resulted in an etoposide-resistant phenotype in neuroendocrine BON cells [Weylandt, Nebrig, et al., 2007], the data presented here are consistent with the proposed role of ClC-3 in vesicular acidification. ClC-7, which locates mainly to the lysosomal compartment, has not been linked to drug resistance so far. However, considering its regulatory function, a similar role in drug resistance as proposed for ClC-3 would be possible. The data presented here therefore suggest that increased vesicular acidity and, thus, etoposide resistance in the concanamycin A-selected LCC-18 cell line, could be due to up-regulation of ClC-3 and/or ClC-7. This interpretation is further supported by the observation that ABC transporters were not up-regulated in our cell line on the mRNA level.

## 4.2 LCC-18 resistant to 1µM etoposide

### 4.2.1 Vesicular acidity and etoposide resistance

In a second experimental approach an etoposide-resistant LCC-18 cell line was created by exposing cells directly to etoposide, and the acidity of intracellular compartments in this resistant cell line was assessed. In accordance with our hypothesis we could show that LCC-18 cells resistant to etoposide had an increased vesicular acidity.

While this data pointed to the proposal that altered pH homeostasis contributed to drug resistance, several limitations of such an interpretation had to be considered. It is likely that tumour cells react not only with one but several protective mechanisms to drug exposure and that, consequently, not one but several systems contribute to drug resistance, even if their importance may differ [Stavrovskaya, 2000]. While little research has been undertaken to investigate the role of vesicular acidity in etoposide resistance, it has widely been described as a substrate of ABC transporters. Consequently, qPCR experiments were performed in analogy to those described for the concanamycin A-selected cell line to understand the molecular basis of etoposide resistance in this cell line.

### 4.2.2 Gene expression

In contrast to the studies in the concanamycin A-selected cell line, the etoposide-resistant cell line showed an enhanced expression of the ABC transporters ABCB4, ABCC1 and ABCC3. The highest level of up-regulation was observed for ABCB4. This transporter functions as phosphatidylcholine flippase in the liver, and mutations can cause progressive familial intrahepatic cholestasis [Szakács, 2006]. Although no data for a potential role in clinical drug resistance has been found, in vitro investigation showed that ABCB4 could promote transcellular transport of several Pgp substrates and could contribute to resistance to taxanes and vinca alkaloids [Smith, 2000; Lage, 2008]. However, no evidence for a participation in resistance to epipodophyllotoxins has been given so far, and the extent to which it contributed to the evolution of etoposide resistance in the LCC-18 cell line is therefore questionable.

ABCC1 together with ABCB1 and ABCG2 belong to the most commonly expressed transporters in multidrug resistance [Sharom, 2008]. ABCC1 is an ubiquitously localised transporter that protects cells against a broad variety of xeno- and endobiotics. Its spectrum includes folates, anthracyclines, vinca-alkaloids, antiandrogens, glutathione- and glucuronide conjugates, organic anions and heavy metals [Munoz, 2007; Borst, 2000]. Etoposide has also been described as its substrate. ABCC3, despite close structural similarity to ABCC1, covers a narrower spectrum and is less commonly expressed. High levels of ABCC3 expression are mainly found in the liver, kidneys and gut, and participation in drug resistance seems to be limited to epipodophyllotoxins and methotrexate [Kool, 1999; Kruh, 2001; Borst, 2000; Lage, 2008]. Since etoposide is substrate of both ABCC1 and ABCC3, their up-regulation could have contributed to drug resistance in the etoposide-resistant cell line used here. It should, nonetheless, be taken into account that mRNA expression was only slightly increased and that we do not know whether this led to a corresponding increase in actual protein expression.

ABCB1 holds an outstanding place among the ABC transporters by conferring the strongest resistance to the widest variety of xenobiotics, including etoposide. Predominantly located at epithelial barriers of the liver, kidney and gastrointestinal tract, it has been shown to be intrinsically over-expressed in tumours of these tissues and to confer a multidrug-resistant phenotype [Szakács, 2006; Lange, 2008; Ambudkar, 2000]. While its abundant participation in drug resistance made it a predominant candidate for resistance in the cell line used here, no up-regulation of ABCB1 could be observed in qPCR. This finding does not exclude a recruitment of ABCB1 by mechanisms other than elevated gene expression. Yagüe et al. showed, for instance, that mRNA expression of ABCB1 did not necessarily correlate with protein expression in the leukemic tumour cell line K562. In their model, stabilisation of mRNA and relief of a translational block but not transcriptional up-regulation were responsible for drug resistance [Yagüe, 2003].

While strongest evidence for participation in etoposide resistance has been given for ABCB1, C1 and C3 [Gaj, 1998; Zelcer, 2001; Allen, 2003; Ambudkar,

## DISCUSSION

1999; Grant, 2008; Szakács, 2006], etoposide has also been described as a potential target of ABCB2, ABCC2, ABCC6 and ABCG2 [Szakács, 2006; Lange, 2008]. Especially ABCG2 is broadly associated with MDR, and Allen et al. showed that it could also confer an etoposide-resistant phenotype in vitro. However, in vivo ABCB1 rather than ABCG2 was responsible for drug resistance in their study [Allen, 2003]. While ABCB2 and the thus far poorly understood transporter ABCC6 conferred only mild resistance to etoposide in transfection models [Izquierdo, 1996; Belinsky, 2002], decreased sensitivity due to ABCC2 was remarkable [König, 1999]. Although we did not investigate the expression of these less commonly explored transporters, their participation would also be possible in our model.

We did not observe any over-expression of ClC-channels or the v-ATPase in LCC-18 resistant to etoposide. Consequently, the qPCR data from the etoposide-resistant cell line points to detoxification by ABC transporters rather than by enhanced vesicular acidification. However, such an interpretation should be viewed in light of the following considerations. Gómez-Martinez et al. showed, for example, that transcriptional up-regulation of ABCB1 in colon carcinoma cell lines did not entail an enhanced protein expression due to translational control [Gómez-Martinez, 2008]. Moreover, an overexpression of ABC transporters could explain etoposide resistance, but does not account for increased compartmental acidification as assessed in the FACS experiments. Increased acidification might be achieved by mechanisms other than up-regulation of ClC-channels or the v-ATPase. Other transporters such as, for example, $Na^+/H^+$-exchangers participate in vesicular pH homeostasis [Faundez, 2004]. It has also been shown that the currents through ClC-channels can be modulated by voltage, extra- and intracellular anions, pH, extracellular $Ca^{2+}$, cell swelling and phosphorylation [Jentsch, Poët, et al., 2005]. Enhanced chloride currents or modified translational control might thus suffice to decrease compartmental pH. Other possibilities for increased vesicular acidification include closure of proton leak pathways of compartmental membranes or modified activity of the v-ATPase [Dutzler, 2004; Torigoe, 2002].

## 4.3 Conclusion

In summary, our data point to an involvement of vesicular acidification in etoposide resistance. In both cell lines a decreased compartmental pH was closely connected to drug resistance. Investigation of the concanamycin A-selected cell line supported a potential role of ClC-3 and ClC-7 in the acquisition of an etoposide-resistant phenotype. The data suggested that mRNA up-regulation of ClC-channels took place as a response to impaired acidification, and might contribute to a drug resistant phenotype in vitro. Conversely, exploration of gene expression in the etoposide-selected cell line indicated that cells reacted to etoposide exposure with an overexpression of ABC transporters and not with an up-regulation of proteins involved in vesicular acidification: we could not observe an up-regulation of the v-ATPase or ClC-channels due to etoposide treatment. However, as interpretation of the expression of mRNA is restricted by several limitations, further explorations are now necessary for a proper understanding of the role of vesicular acidity and ClC-channels in drug resistance. These may, for instance, include a screening of tissue samples for the expression of ClC-channels. Considering the lack of available antibodies for the channels, the qPCR assay established here would in this context constitute an easily applicable tool for the investigation of a potential participation of the ClC-channels in drug resistance in vivo. Other explorations might include the direct pharmacological targeting of ClC-channels in functional cell experiments or an investigation of ClC-channels' protein expression in drug resistant cell lines based on Western Blotting.

# 5 Abstract

Drug resistance constitutes a major challenge in the treatment of metastatic neuroendocrine cancer. Chemotherapeutic regimes for these tumours employ weak-base drugs including, for instance, etoposide. Especially for this medication, a mechanism of resistance was suggested that linked increased acidification of intracellular compartments to the evolution of drug resistance. Chloride channels of the ClC-family play a pivotal role in the pH homeostasis of cellular organelles, and recently the first evidence for a potential role of ClC-3 in drug resistance was given.

Following this finding, our work aimed to further elucidate the role of ClC-channels and compartmental acidification in the evolution of etoposide resistance. In this context we focused on the question of whether an up-regulation of intracellular ClC-channels could be observed as a cellular response to chemotherapeutic drugs and whether it would entail increased compartmental acidity and thus contribute to the evolution of drug resistance in vitro. We addressed the problem through two different experimental approaches.

In a first approach, cells of the neuroendocrine tumour cell line LCC-18 were selected by long-term exposure to the v-ATPase inhibitor concanamycin A and etoposide sensitivity was assessed as a function of altered pH homeostasis. In these experiments we could show that intracellular compartments were, indeed, more acidic due to concanamycin A selection and that the selected cells were also more resistant to etoposide. Moreover, exploration of gene expression by qPCR supported a potential role of ClC-3 and ClC-7 in the acquisition of an etoposide-resistant phenotype. Our data suggested that mRNA up-regulation of ClC-channels might entail increased vesicular acidification and contribute to a drug resistant phenotype.

In a second approach, LCC-18 cells were selected for etoposide resistance, and compartmental acidity was assessed as a function of etoposide resistance. In the etoposide-resistant cell line intracellular compartments were also more acidic than in control cells, and this data pointed to a contribution of enhanced vesicular acidity to etoposide resistance. However, genetic investigation indicated that in these cells overexpression of ABC transporters let to the resistant phenotype: we could not observe any up-regulation of ClC-channels due to etoposide treatment. As interpretation of mRNA expression faces several limitations, further explorations are now necessary for a proper understanding of the role of vesicular acidity and ClC-channels in drug resistance.

# 6 References

Allen, J.D., Van Dort, S.C., Buitelaar, M., van Tellingen, O., and Schinkel, A.H. (2003). Mouse breast cancer resistance protein (Bcrp1/Abcg2) mediates etoposide resistance and transport, but etoposide oral availability is limited primarily by P-glycoprotein. *Cancer Res*, **63**:1339-344.

Altan, N., Chen, Y., Schindler, M., and Simon, S.M. (1998). Defective acidification in human breast tumor cells and implications for chemotherapy. *J Exp Med*, **187**:1583-598.

Altan, N., Chen, Y., Schindler, M., and Simon, S.M. (1999). Tamoxifen inhibits acidification in cells independent of the estrogen receptor. *Proc Natl Acad Sci USA*, **96**:4432-37.

Ambudkar, S.V., Dey, S., Hrycyna, C.A., Ramachandra, M., Pastan, I., and Gottesman, M.M. (1999). Biochemical, cellular, and pharmacological aspects of the multidrug transporter. *Annu Rev Pharmacol Toxicol*, **39**:361-398.

Arnold, R. (2005). Endocrine tumours of the gastrointestinal tract. Introduction: definition, historical aspects, classification, staging, prognosis and therapeutic options. *Best Pract Res Clin Gastroenterol*, **19**:491-505.

Belinsky, M.G., Chen, Z.S., Shchaveleva, I., Zeng, H., and Kruh, G.D. (2002). Characterization of the drug resistance and transport properties of multidrug resistance protein 6 (MRP6, ABCC6). *Cancer Res*, **62**:6172-77.

Borst, P., Evers, R., Kool, M., and Wijnholds, J. (2000). A family of drug transporters: the multidrug resistance-associated proteins. *J Natl Cancer Inst*, **92**:1295-1302.

Bowman, E.J., Graham, L.A., Stevens, T.H., and Bowman, B.J. (2004). The bafilomycin/concanamycin binding site in subunit c of the V-ATPases from Neurospora crassa and Saccharomyces cerevisiae. *J Biol Chem*, **279**:33131-38.

Bustin, S.A. (2000). Absolute quantification of mRNA using real-time reverse transcription polymerase chain reaction assays. *J Mol Endocrinol*, **25**:169-193.

Bustin, S.A., and Nolan, T. (2004). Pitfalls of quantitative real-time reverse-transcription polymerase chain reaction. *J Biomol Tech*, **15**:155-166.

Champaneria, M.C., Modlin, I.M., Kidd, M., and Eick, G.N. (2006). Friedrich Feyrter: A Precise Intellect in a Diffuse System. *Neuroendocrinology*, **83**:394-404.

Creutzfeldt, W. (1996). Carcinoid tumors: development of our knowledge. *World J Surg*, **20**:126-131.

Czaplinski, K., and Singer, R.H. (2006). Pathways for mRNA localization in the cytoplasm. *Trends Biochem Sci*, **31**:687-693.

Dutzler, R. (2007). A structural perspective on ClC channel and transporter function. *FEBS Lett*, **581**:2839-844.

Faundez, V., and Hartzell, H.C. (2004). Intracellular chloride channels: determinants of function in the endosomal pathway. *Sci STKE*, **233**:re8.

Gaj, C.L., Anyanwutaku, I., Chang, Y.H., and Cheng, Y.C. (1998). Decreased drug accumulation without increased drug efflux in a novel MRP-overexpressing multidrug-resistant cell line. *Biochem Pharmacol*, **55**:1199-1211.

Grant, C.E., Gao, M., DeGorter, M.K., Cole, S.P., and Deeley, R.G. (2008). Structural determinants of substrate specificity differences between human multidrug resistance protein (MRP) 1 (ABCC1) and MRP3 (ABCC3). *Drug Metab Dispos*, **36**:2571-581.

Gómez-Martínez, A., García-Morales, P., Carrato, A., Castro-Galache, M., Soto, J., Carrasco-García, E., et al. (2007). Post-transcriptional Regulation of P-Glycoprotein Expression in Cancer Cell Lines. *Mol Cancer Res*, **5(6)**:641-53.

Hara-Chikuma, M., Yang, B., Sonawane, N.D., Sasaki, S., Uchida, S., and Verkman, A.S. (2005). ClC-3 chloride channels facilitate endosomal acidification and chloride accumulation. *J Biol Chem*, **280**:1241-47.

Huggett, J., Dheda, K., Bustin, S., and Zumla, A. (2005). Real-time RT-PCR normalisation; strategies and considerations. *Genes Immun*, **6**:279-284.

Izquierdo, M.A., Neefjes, J.J., Mathari, A.E., Flens, M.J., Scheffer, G.L., and Scheper, R.J. (1996). Overexpression of the ABC transporter TAP in multidrug-resistant human cancer cell lines. *Br J Cancer*, **74**:1961-67.

# REFERENCES

Izumi, H., Torigoe, T., Ishiguchi, H., Uramoto, H., Yoshida, Y., Tanabe, M., Ise, T., Murakami, T., Yoshida, T., et al. (2003). Cellular pH regulators: potentially promising molecular targets for cancer chemotherapy. *Cancer Treat Rev*, **29**:541-49.

Jacquet, E., Girard, J.M., Ramaen, O., Pamlard, O., Lévaique, H., Betton, J.M., Dassa, E., and Chesneau, O. (2008). ATP hydrolysis and pristinamycin IIA inhibition of the Staphylococcus aureus Vga(A), a dual ABC protein involved in streptogramin A resistance. *J Biol Chem*, **283**:25332-39.

Jentsch, T.J., Neagoe, I., and Scheel, O. (2005). CLC chloride channels and transporters. *Curr Opin Neurobiol*, **15**:319-325.

Jentsch, T.J., Poët, M., Fuhrmann, J.C., and Zdebik, A.A. (2005). Physiological functions of CLC Cl-channels gleaned from human genetic disease and mouse models. *Annu Rev Physiol*, **67**:779-807.

Jentsch, T.J., Steinmeyer, K., and Schwarz, G. (1990). Primary structure of Torpedo marmorata chloride channel isolated by expression cloning in Xenopus oocytes. *Nature*, **348**:510-14.

Kasper, D., Planells-Cases, R., Fuhrmann, J.C., Scheel, O., Zeitz, O., Ruether, K., Schmitt, A., Poët, M., Steinfeld, R., et al. (2005). Loss of the chloride channel ClC-7 leads to lysosomal storage disease and neurodegeneration. *EMBO J*, **24**:1079-091.

Klöppel, G. (2007). Tumour biology and histopathology of neuroendocrine tumours. *Best Pract Res Clin Endocrinol Metab*, **21**:15-31.

Klöppel, G., and Anlauf, M. (2005). Epidemiology, tumour biology and histopathological classification of neuroendocrine tumours of the gastrointestinal tract. *Best Pract Res Clin Gastroenterol*, **19**:507-517.

Kool, M., van der Linden, M., de Haas, M., Scheffer, G.L., de Vree, J.M., Smith, A.J., Jansen, G., Peters, G.J., Ponne, N., et al. (1999). MRP3, an organic anion transporter able to transport anti-cancer drugs. *Proc Natl Acad Sci USA*, **96**:6914-19.

König, J., Nies, A.T., Cui, Y., Leier, I., and Keppler, D. (1999). Conjugate export pumps of the multidrug resistance protein (MRP) family: localization, substrate specificity, and MRP2-mediated drug resistance. *Biochim Biophys Acta*, **1461**:377-394.

Kruh, G.D., Zeng, H., Rea, P.A., Liu, G., Chen, Z.S., Lee, K., and Belinsky, M.G. (2001). MRP subfamily transporters and resistance to anticancer agents. *J Bioenerg Biomembr*, **33**:493-501.

Lage, H. (2008). An overview of cancer multidrug resistance: a still unsolved problem. *Cell Mol Life Sci*, **65**:3145-167.

Li, X., Wang, T., Zhao, Z., and Weinman, S.A. (2002). The ClC-3 chloride channel promotes acidification of lysosomes in CHO-K1 and Huh-7 cells. *Am J Physiol Cell Physiol*, **282**:C1483-491.

Lundqvist, M., Mark, J., Funa, K., Heldin, N.E., Morstyn, G., Wedell, B., Layton, J., and Oberg, K. (1991). Characterisation of a cell line (LCC-18) from a cultured human neuroendocrine-differentiated colonic carcinoma. *Eur J Cancer*, **27**:1663-68.

Meresse, P., Dechaux, E., Monneret, C., and Bertounesque, E. (2004). Etoposide: discovery and medicinal chemistry. *Curr Med Chem*, **11**:2443-466.

Millot, C., Millot, J.M., Morjani, H., Desplaces, A., and Manfait, M. (1997). Characterization of acidic vesicles in multidrug-resistant and sensitive cancer cells by acridine orange staining and confocal microspectrofluorometry. *J Histochem Cytochem*, **45**:1255-264.

Modlin, I.M., Champaneria, M.C., Bornschein, J., and Kidd, M. (2006). Evolution of the diffuse neuroendocrine system--clear cells and cloudy origins. *Neuroendocrinology*, **84**:69-82.

Moertel, C.G., Kvols, L.K., O'Connell, M.J., and Rubin, J. (1991). Treatment of neuroendocrine carcinomas with combined etoposide and cisplatin. Evidence of major therapeutic activity in the anaplastic variants of these neoplasms. *Cancer*, **68**:227-232.

Moore, M.J. (2005). From birth to death: the complex lives of eukaryotic mRNAs. *Science*, **309**:1514-18.

Moriyama, Y., Manabe, T., Yoshimori, T., Tashiro, Y., and Futai, M. (1994). ATP-dependent uptake of anti-neoplastic agents by acidic organelles. *J Biochem*, **115**:213-18.

Munoz, M., Henderson, M., Haber, M., and Norris, M. (2007). Role of the MRP1/ABCC1 multidrug transporter protein in cancer. *IUBMB Life*, **59**:752-57.

Nishi, T., and Forgac, M. (2002). The vacuolar (H+)-ATPases--nature's most versatile proton pumps. *Nat Rev Mol Cell Biol*, **3**:94-103.

O'Toole, D., Hentic, O., Corcos, O., and Ruszniewski, P. (2004). Chemotherapy for gastro-enteropancreatic endocrine tumours. *Neuroendocrinology*, **80**(Suppl.1): 79-84.

Olsen, M.L., Schade, S., Lyons, S.A., Amaral, M.D., and Sontheimer, H. (2003). Expression of voltage-gated chloride channels in human glioma cells. *J Neurosci*, **23**:5572-582.

# REFERENCES

Ouar, Z., Bens, M., Vignes, C., Paulais, M., Pringel, C., Fleury, J., Cluzeaud, F., Lacave, R., and Vandewalle, A. (2003). Inhibitors of vacuolar H+-ATPase impair the preferential accumulation of daunomycin in lysosomes and reverse the resistance to anthracyclines in drug-resistant renal epithelial cells. *Biochem J,* **370**:185-193.

Pearse, A.G. (1969). The cytochemistry and ultrastructure of polypeptide hormone-producing cells of the APUD series and the embryologic, physiologic and pathologic implications of the concept. *J Histochem Cytochem,* **17**:303-313.

Pearse, A.G. (1977). The diffuse endocrine (paracine) system: Feyrter's concept and its modern history. *Verh Dtsch Ges Pathol,* **61**:2-6.

Plöckinger, U., and Wiedenmann, B. (2005). Endocrine tumours of the gastrointestinal tract. Management of metastatic endocrine tumours. *Best Pract Res Clin Gastroenterol,* **19**:553-576.

Plöckinger, U., Rindi, G., Arnold, R., Eriksson, B., Krenning, E.P., de Herder, W.W., Goede, A., Caplin, M., Oberg, K., et al. (2004). Guidelines for the diagnosis and treatment of neuroendocrine gastrointestinal tumours. A consensus statement on behalf of the European Neuroendocrine Tumour Society (ENETS). *Neuroendocrinology,* **80**:394-424.

Raghunand, N., and Gillies, R.J. (2000). pH and drug resistance in tumors. *Drug Resist Updat,* **3**:39-47.

Raghunand, N., Martínez-Zaguilán, R., Wright, S.H., and Gillies, R.J. (1999). pH and drug resistance. II. Turnover of acidic vesicles and resistance to weakly basic chemotherapeutic drugs. *Biochem Pharmacol,* **57**:1047-058.

Rajagopal, A., and Simon, S.M. (2003). Subcellular localization and activity of multidrug resistance proteins. *Mol Biol Cell,* **14**:3389-399.

Rindi, G., and Klöppel, G. (2004). Endocrine tumors of the gut and pancreas tumor biology and classification. *Neuroendocrinology,* **80**(Suppl.1):12-15.

Rindi, G., Klöppel, G., Alhman, H., Caplin, M., Couvelard, A., de Herder, W.W., Erikssson, B., Falchetti, A., Falconi, M., et al. (2006). TNM staging of foregut (neuro)endocrine tumors: a consensus proposal including a grading system. *Virchows Arch,* **449**:395-401.

Roos, A. (1978). Weak acids, weak bases and intracellular pH. *Respir Physiol,* **33**:27-30.

Rougemaille, M., Villa, T., Gudipati, R.K., and Libri, D. (2008). mRNA journey to the cytoplasm: attire required. *Biol Cell,* **100**:327-342.

Schindler, M., Grabski, S., Hoff, E., and Simon, S.M. (1996). Defective pH regulation of acidic compartments in human breast cancer cells (MCF-7) is normalized in adriamycin-resistant cells (MCF-7adr). *Biochemistry,* **35**:2811-17.

Sennoune, S.R., Luo, D., and Martínez-Zaguilán, R. (2004). Plasmalemmal vacuolar-type H+-ATPase in cancer biology. *Cell Biochem Biophys,* **40**:185-206.

Sharom, F.J. (2008). ABC multidrug transporters: structure, function and role in chemoresistance. *Pharmacogenomics,* **9**:105-127.

Shyu, A.B., Wilkinson, M.F., and van Hoof, A. (2008). Messenger RNA regulation: to translate or to degrade. *EMBO J,* **27**:471-481.

Simon, S., Roy, D., and Schindler, M. (1994). Intracellular pH and the control of multidrug resistance. *Proc Natl Acad Sci USA,* **91**:1128-132.

Simon, S.M., and Schindler, M. (1994). Cell biological mechanisms of multidrug resistance in tumors. *Proc Natl Acad Sci USA,* **91**:3497-3504.

Smith, A.J., van Helvoort, A., van Meer, G., Szabo, K., Welker, E., Szakacs, G., Varadi, A., Sarkadi, B., and Borst, P. (2000). MDR3 P-glycoprotein, a phosphatidylcholine translocase, transports several cytotoxic drugs and directly interacts with drugs as judged by interference with nucleotide trapping. *J Biol Chem,* **275**:23530-39.

Smith, A.N., Lovering, R.C., Futai, M., Takeda, J., Brown, D., and Karet, F.E. (2003). Revised nomenclature for mammalian vacuolar-type H+ -ATPase subunit genes. *Mol Cell,* **12**:801-03.

Stavrovskaya, A.A. (2000). Cellular mechanisms of multidrug resistance of tumor cells. *Biochemistry (Mosc),* **65**:95-106.

Suh, K.S., and Yuspa, S.H. (2005). Intracellular chloride channels: critical mediators of cell viability and potential targets for cancer therapy. *Curr Pharm Des 11,* 2753-764.

Sun-Wada, G.H., Wada, Y., and Futai, M. (2004). Diverse and essential roles of mammalian vacuolar-type proton pump ATPase: toward the physiological understanding of inside acidic compartments. *Biochim Biophys Acta,* **1658**:106-114.

# REFERENCES

Szakács, G., Paterson, J.K., Ludwig, J.A., Booth-Genthe, C., and Gottesman, M.M. (2006). Targeting multidrug resistance in cancer. *Nat Rev Drug Discov,* **5**:219-234.

Taal, B.G., and Visser, O. (2004). Epidemiology of neuroendocrine tumours. *Neuroendocrinology,* **80**(Suppl.1):3-7.

Torigoe, T., Izumi, H., Ise, T., Murakami, T., Uramoto, H., Ishiguchi, H., Yoshida, Y., Tanabe, M., Nomoto, M., and Kohno, K. (2002). Vacuolar H(+)-ATPase: functional mechanisms and potential as a target for cancer chemotherapy. *Anticancer Drugs,* **13**:237-243.

Ursos, L.M., Dzekunov, S.M., and Roepe, P.D. (2000). The effects of chloroquine and verapamil on digestive vacuolar pH of P. falciparum either sensitive or resistant to chloroquine. *Mol Biochem Parasitol,* **110**:125-134.

Valencia-Sanchez, M.A., Liu, J., Hannon, G.J., and Parker, R. (2006). Control of translation and mRNA degradation by miRNAs and siRNAs. *Genes Dev,* **20**:515-524.

Van Maanen, J.M., Retèl, J., de Vries, J., and Pinedo, H.M. (1988). Mechanism of action of antitumor drug etoposide: a review. *J Natl Cancer Inst,* **80**:1526-533.

Vandesompele, J., De Preter, K., Pattyn, F., Poppe, B., Van Roy, N., De Paepe, A., and Speleman, F. (2002). Accurate normalization of real-time quantitative RT-PCR data by geometric averaging of multiple internal control genes. *Genome Biol,* **3**:RESEARCH0034.

Weylandt, K.H., Nebrig, M., Jansen-Rosseck, N., Amey, J.S., Carmena, D., Wiedenmann, B., Higgins, C.F., and Sardini, A. (2007). ClC-3 expression enhances etoposide resistance by increasing acidification of the late endocytic compartment. *Mol Cancer Ther,* **6**:979-986.

Williams, E.D., and Sandler, M. (1963). The classification of carcinoid tumours. *Lancet,* **1**:238-39.

Yague, E., Armesilla, A.L., Harrison, G., Elliott, J., Sardini, A., Higgins, C.F., and Raguz, S. (2003). P-glycoprotein (MDR1) expression in leukemic cells is regulated at two distinct steps, mRNA stabilization and translational initiation. *J Biol Chem,* **278**:10344-352.

Zelcer, N., Saeki, T., Reid, G., Beijnen, J.H., and Borst, P. (2001). Characterization of drug transport by the human multidrug resistance protein 3 (ABCC3). *J Biol Chem,* **276**:46400-07.

Zifarelli, G., and Pusch, M. (2007). CLC chloride channels and transporters: a biophysical and physiological perspective. *Rev Physiol Biochem Pharmacol,* **158**:23-76.

# Appendix

## List of Abbreviations

| | |
|---|---|
| ABC transporters | Adenosine triphosphate binding cassette transporters |
| AO | Acridine orange |
| APUD | Amine precursor uptake and decarboxylation |
| ATP | Adenosine triphosphate |
| Cl- | Chloride |
| cm | Centimetre |
| DMSO | Dimethyl Sulfoxide |
| FACS | Fluorescence activated cell sorting |
| FBS | Fetal bovine serum |
| GEP-NET | Gastroenteropancreatic neuroendocrine tumours |
| GFP | Green fluorescent protein |
| HPRT1 | Hypoxanthine phosphoribosyltransferase 1 |
| MDR | Multi drug resistance |
| µl | Microlitre |
| ml | Millilitre |
| µM | Micromolar |
| mosm | Milliosmol |
| ng | Nanogram |
| nm | Nanometre |
| nM | Nanomolar |
| NET | Neuroendocrine tumours |
| PBS | Phosphate buffered saline |
| PCR | Polymerase chain reaction |
| qPCR | Quantitative real time polymerase chain reaction |
| RPLP0 | Large ribosomal protein P0 |
| RT reaction | Reverse transcriptase reaction |
| TBP | TATA binding protein |
| v-($H^+$)-ATPase | Vacuolar (proton) adenosine triphosphate |
| WHO | World health organisation |

APPENDIX

# List of Tables and Figures

**Figure 1:** Role of ClC-channels in the regulation of vesicular acidification   10
**Figure 2:** FACS assay of LCC-18 resistant to 1nM concanamycin A   25
**Figure 3:** Cell proliferation assay of LCC-18 resistant to 1nM concanamycin A   26
**Figure 4:** Gene expression of LCC-18 resistant to 1nM concanamycin A   30
**Figure 5:** Cell proliferation assay of LCC-18 resistant to 1µM etoposide   31
**Figure 6:** FACS assay of LCC-18 resistant to 1µM etoposide   32
**Figure 7:** Gene expression of LCC-18 resistant to 1µM etoposide   34


**Table 1:** Criteria for assessing the prognosis of neuroendocrine tumours of the gastrointestinal tract   5
**Table 2:** Subunits of the v-ATPase   9
**Table 3:** Function and localisation of mammalian ClC-channels   12
**Table 4:** Reaction mixture for RT reaction   19
**Table 5:** Procedure for primer design   20
**Table 6:** Sequences of qPCR primers   21
**Table 7:** Reaction mixture for qPCR   22
**Table 8:** Cycling conditions for qPCR   22
**Table 9:** M-value and physiological function of control genes   29

APPENDIX

# Zusammenfassung

Chemotherapieresistenz stellt eine wesenliche Herausforderung in der Behandlung von metastasierten, neuroendokrinen Tumoren dar. Therapiepläne dieser Tumore beinhalten schwach basische Medikamente wie zum Beispiel Etoposid. Für diese Medikamentengruppe wurde ein Resistenzmechanismus vorgeschlagen, der auf einer erhöhten Azidifizierung intrazellulärer Kompartimente beruht. Chlorid Kanäle der ClC-Familie spielen eine Schlüsselrolle in der pH-Homeostase intrazellulärer Organellen und kürzlich wurde erstmals eine mögliche Beteiligung von ClC-3 bei Chemotherapieresistenz gezeigt.

Die vorliegende Arbeit hat in diesem Rahmen ein besseres Verständnis der Rolle von ClC-Kanälen und kompartmentaler Azidifizierung bei der Entstehung von Arzneimittelresistenz zum Ziel. Wir konzentrierten uns dabei auf die Fragen, ob eine Hochregulierung von intrazellulären ClC-Kanälen als zelluläre Antwort auf Chemotherapeutika beobachtet werden kann und ob eine solche Hochregulierung tatsächlich eine erhöhte vesikuläre Azidität nach sich ziehen und so zur Evolution von Chemotherapieresistenz in vitro beitragen kann. Die Fragestellungen wurden mittels zwei komplementärer Ansätze untersucht.

In einem ersten Versuchsansatz wurden Zellen der neuroendokrinen Tumorzelllinie LCC-18 durch langfristige Exposition zu dem v-ATPase Inhibitor Concanamycin A selektiert und dann auf ihre Etoposidresistenz in Abhängigkeit von der veränderten intravesikulären pH-Homeostase untersucht. Wir konnten zeigen, dass intrazelluläre Kompartimente in der Concanamycin A-resistenten Zellinie in der Tat azidischer als in Kontrollzellen waren und dass die Zellen ebenfalls resistenter gegen Etoposid waren. Darüberhinaus deutete die Untersuchung der Genexpression mittels quantitativer Polymerasen Kettenreaktion auf eine mögliche Rolle von ClC-3 und ClC-7 bei der Entstehung des Etoposid-resistenten Phänotyps hin. Diese Daten legten nahe, dass mRNA-Hochregulierung von ClC-Kanälen eine erhöhte vesikuläre Azidifizierung nach sich ziehen und so zu einem chemotherapieresistenten Phänotyp beitragen kann.

In einem zweiten Versuchsansatz wurden LCC-18 Zellen unter langzeitiger Gabe von Etoposid selektiert und die kompartimentale Azidizität in Abhängigkeit von dem Etoposid-resistenten Phänotyp untersucht. In der Etoposid-resistenten Zelllinie fanden sich azidischere intrazelluläre Kompartimente als in Kontrollzellen. Anders als in den Concanamycin A-selektieren Zellen legte die genetische Untersuchung mittels Polymerasen Kettenreaktion jedoch nahe, dass die Etoposid-selektierten Zellen mit einer Überexpression von ABC-Transportern und nicht mit einer Hochregulierung von Kontrollmechanismen des vesikulären pH-Wertes auf die Etoposidexposition reagierten. Wir konnnten dementsprechend keine Hochregulierung von ClC-Kanälen in Folge von einer Etoposidbehandlung beobachten. Da die Interpretation der mRNA-Expression jedoch verschiedenen Einschränkungen unterliegt, sind nun weitere Untersuchungen für ein angemessenes Verständnis der Rolle von vesikulärer Azidifizierung und ClC-Kanälen bei Chemotherapieresistenz notwendig.

## Acknowledgments

Many people have helped me realize this project, and I am deeply grateful for all the moral and material support that I was lucky to receive. First and foremost I would like to thank my supervisors Alessandro Sardini from the Membrane Transport Group of the MRC Clinical Sciences Centre in London and Karsten Weylandt from the Medizinische Klinik mit Schwerpunkt Hepatologie und Gastroenterologie der Medizinischen Fakultät Charite – Universitätsmedizin Berlin. In addition to having made possible my exchange between their institutions, Drs. Sardini and Weylandt advised me closely and remained truly available until the project was finished. I deeply appreciate their great support.

At the Clinical Sciences Centre I am deeply indebted to the former Membrane Transport Group, led by Christopher Higgins, who accepted me as member of their team and introduced me to laboratory research. I would especially like to thank Selina Raguz for guiding me through the difficulties of qPCR and David Carmena for his friendship and cheerful advice in many difficult moments of my project. Within the framework of the Membrane Transport Group I am lucky to have been provided with both the kind and necessary guidance to find my way, as well as the freedom to follow my own tentative interests within the field of ClC-channels and drug resistance.

I am very grateful to the German Academic Exchange Service and the German National Academic Foundation for their financial support without which the project would never have been possible.

Last but not least I would like to thank my friends and my family for always listening to my ups and downs and for supporting me steadily through all the stages of my thesis. In the last phase special thanks to Jane Cheng for helping me with many details and for proof-reading the entire document, and to Hilary and Mariel Finucane for their statistical advice.

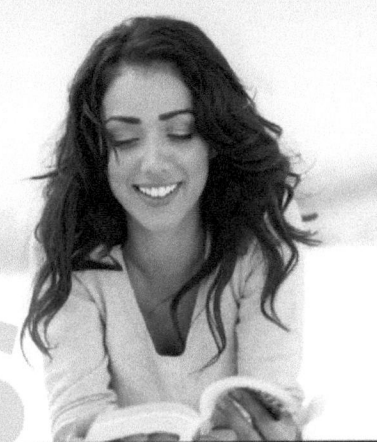
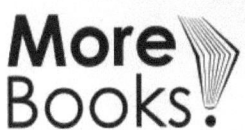

# I want morebooks!

Buy your books fast and straightforward online - at one of world's fastest growing online book stores! Environmentally sound due to Print-on-Demand technologies.

Buy your books online at
**www.morebooks.shop**

Kaufen Sie Ihre Bücher schnell und unkompliziert online – auf einer der am schnellsten wachsenden Buchhandelsplattformen weltweit! Dank Print-On-Demand umwelt- und ressourcenschonend produziert.

Bücher schneller online kaufen
**www.morebooks.shop**

KS OmniScriptum Publishing
Brivibas gatve 197
LV-1039 Riga, Latvia
Telefax: +371 686 204 55

info@omniscriptum.com
www.omniscriptum.com

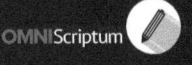

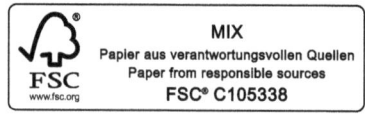

Printed by Books on Demand GmbH, Norderstedt / Germany